Patriarchy, Misogyny and *Breastfeeding*

SUSANNA I. SCURRY

Copyright © 2024 by Susanna I. Scurry.

Library of Congress Control Number:		2023922257
ISBN:	Hardcover	979-8-3694-9428-8
	Softcover	979-8-3694-9427-1
	eBook	979-8-3694-9429-5

All rights reserved. No part of this book may be reproduced or transmitted in any form or by any means, electronic or mechanical, including photocopying, recording, or by any information storage and retrieval system, without permission in writing from the copyright owner.

Any people depicted in stock imagery provided by Getty Images are models, and such images are being used for illustrative purposes only.
Certain stock imagery © Getty Images.

Print information available on the last page.

Rev. date: 08/15/2024

To order additional copies of this book, contact:
Xlibris
AU TFN: 1 800 844 927 (Toll Free inside Australia)
AU Local: (02) 8310 8187 (+61 2 8310 8187 from outside Australia)
www.Xlibris.com.au
Orders@Xlibris.com.au
854342

Contents

Introduction vii

1	My Story	1
2	Breastfeeding as a Human Rights Issue	23
3	A History of Birthing	42
4	The Changing Nature of Birthing	62
5	The Baby-Friendly Hospital Initiative	83
6	The Neo-Baby Friendly Hospital Initiative	94
7	A History of Infant Feeding	113
8	The Unique Qualities of Breastmilk	126
9	The Economics of Breastfeeding	136
10	Improving Breastfeeding Rates	153
11	EQUIP: A continuity of care randomised control trial pilot research study	175
12	Discussion and Conclusion	185

References 197
Acknowledgements 215

Introduction

In the middle of Australia's red centre resides the oldest living culture on earth. There children are taught, in stories known as *chi chi*, the rules of survival. The *Tjukurpa*, or deep knowledge, comes from creation times and helps children understand what is important. They learn to trust their instincts, look after the land and hunt sustainably. They learn that women have an obligation to look after their children, and the right to defend them.

Australia's First Nations people lived sustainably and nurtured the land for more than 65,000 years. When the British colonised Australia to set up penal colonies, there was one white woman for every six men. The harsh beginnings created a brutal environment, and *terra nullius* (land belonging to no one) made the Indigenous people invisible and, as a consequence, destroyed much of the land, flora and fauna. The abuse and exploitation of both Indigenous and white women came with the colonisers and continues to this day.

Most new families say that getting through the birth looms large throughout the pregnancy and takes the focus away from what is to come after the baby is born. They tell me that there is a great emphasis on the baby's wellbeing by health professionals leading up to and when the baby is born. Following the birth, interest in the mother falls away and doctors have little input unless there is a medical reason. Hence, within the hierarchical institutional structures, the dominant power group allows little time for the mother to rest and recover or learn to be a carer for the baby, and how to breastfeed. Looking after a baby can be relentless and tiring, often affecting a women's physical and mental health. As society has evolved and created a global village, the current nuclear family has seen many of the support structures for mothers removed. Many families tell me without support from adequately trained caring health professionals, family and friends, they would have felt very vulnerable after giving birth.

The impetus for undertaking this book is a question I have often pondered. What is it that makes a mother? Intuitively, mammalian mothers would give their lives to protect their children and most women know breastfeeding is the optimum way to feed a baby. Having said this, I am not interested in the breast-versus-bottle debate, which has been used to divide women for decades; a woman's choice is her own business. However, when public monies are being paid for the care of women, they have the right to evidence-based information and education. Whatever the women's choice, she needs to be given the correct information to achieve her feeding goals.

My intention in telling my truth is to share the lessons I have learned throughout my life and career to empower others, and ultimately to bring about changes that will improve the lives of women and their families. When discussing my writings with different people over the many years this book has taken to complete, everyone has a story to tell. But the overarching theme is how hard it is to be a parent.

Birthing has changed throughout history and during my lifetime. My viewpoint will be challenged by others with a different way of knowing, but it has been gained during a long life and my experience as a white female growing up and becoming a mother in Australia. I have birthed five times and fed two children following World Health Organization (WHO) recommendations within the medicalised model, as the result of a lack of adequate breastfeeding education. I became a midwife and lactation consultant because of my experiences, and have assisted my own family and many other women to birth and breastfeed. My role as mother, grandmother, registered nurse, midwife and international board-certified lactation consultant – working within Australia and overseas – gives me a perspective from the bottom-up of how the medicalisation of birth has disempowered women and impacted their journey to motherhood.

A short explanation of patriarchy and misogyny

The subordination of women has been explained historically in a number of ways. One plausible theory is that, as humans evolved males grew bigger, and used their larger size and protective hormones, designed to keep the group safe, to dominate the smaller female.

Angela Saini, in her book exploring the origins of patriarchy (Saini, 2023), believes human societies developed over time and were not always male dominated. Her research into different cultures and historical periods demonstrates that patriarchy came about due to a need to protect the wealth of those in power. As empires began to expand, these ideas spread. In Mesopotamia, 6000-year-old stone tablets list population and resources, and show that the rulers in early agrarian societies needed warriors to protect the wealth of the state. They created rules that required women to produce babies and men to be warriors. The rules perpetuated the myth of male superiority and made women subservient. Those males and females who deviated from what was expected were condemned as unnatural.

In Australia, patriarchy and misogyny was imported with colonialism and imperialism. Feminist writer Anne Summers wrote, 'I do not think we can begin to understand women's position in Australia today, nor men's attitudes to women, without at least a cursory consideration of those past events and ideas which cast shadows on the present' (Summers, 2002).

Between 1788 and 1869, 162,000 prisoners were transported to Australia, and used as free labour until transportation ended. Poor English and Irish women prisoners who had committed crimes of poverty were given harsh penalties and banished to the penal settlement, where they were used and abused as unpaid labourers by those in positions of power. When gold was discovered in 1856, another influx of migrants arrived in search of eureka. In 1912, fearing for Australia's security and economic wellbeing, the Australian Government introduced a baby bonus to encourage white

Australian families to have more children. The 5-pound bonus was aimed at increasing the low white population base of 4 million. In May 2004, the Australian Government again introduced a baby bonus – this time AUS$3000 per child – with subsequent increases to encourage new mothers to have more children. The Australian newspaper reported Federal Treasurer Peter Costello as saying, 'One [baby] for your husband and one for your wife and one for the country' *(The Age*, 2004).

While the Treasurer may have seen the baby bonus as helping families, a one-off payment is short-sighted. If the monies were spent on structural reforms, for example free childcare, women would have improved autonomy. It is a complete nonsense that childcare is not free. If women could work or be educated without the burden of paid childcare they would not be dependant, and structural reforms to support women, which recognise their contribution to the community as well as the burden when taking time to have children, would reflect the physical and emotional burden involved.

1

My Story

I was born on 6 September 1953, the first child before two brothers. My arrival took place in the Walwa Bush Nursing Hospital and was the first birth conducted by the new and only doctor in town. It was uncomplicated and normal, like the births of my two brothers would be. My mother breastfed according to the scientific mothering practices taught at that time, until the doctor recommended boiled cow's milk. She had reported to him at six weeks that I cried frequently, and she thought her milk was inadequate to sustain me. As a consequence she weaned her two sons at the same age.

Early childhood

As a child, I was plagued with constant ear and throat infections and, shortly after commencing school, admitted to hospital with glomerulonephritis, a kidney disease caused by an immunological reaction to repeated streptococcal throat infections in an unlucky few. My parents were prepared for the worst, and I was transferred to the Albury Base Hospital. What I remember about that time was being desperately homesick and missing my parents. They were not allowed to stay in the hospital, and the trip from Walwa to Albury was one and a half hours away on a winding road that followed the Murray River. After some time, I was returned home to the Walwa hospital, where my parents would visit me whenever visiting hours permitted. My class teacher visited most days, bringing books and classwork so I would not fall behind.

The memory of the painful injections of penicillin, twice a day, live with me still. Depression and isolation from my family led to tantrums when my parents left the hospital and eventually forced my parents to negotiate with the hospital staff to bring me home. They said that, if I was not going to survive, they would rather see me happy. An arrangement was made to keep me resting at home, with trips to the hospital for the penicillin injections. I cried when being driven there and begged my parents not to make me have them.

My parents were ingenious and developed strategies to keep me still and quiet at home. They agreed they would buy me a puppy when I got well if I did not 'play up', and acquired Mickey, a green budgerigar. They had me train Mickey by ringing a small bell attached to a little rocking toy. If I remained quiet and still after ringing the bell, Mickey would sometimes fly from his cage to me to receive a sugar treat. Mickey and books were my friends during that time. I have often wondered if my illness could have been prevented had my mother breastfed me for longer.

My parents owned and operated the Tintaldra Hotel, a former customs house beside the bridge that separated Victoria and NSW on the Murray River. Tintaldra is tiny, and I had no friends nearby my own age. When not at school or working in the hotel, I spent hours in the boat or canoe, or swimming and fishing in the river. I lived mainly in my own head and dreamed.

I wanted to train as a vet or archaeologist when I left school. I was often brought featherless birds by patrons at the hotel. The bird's nests were being destroyed as the trees from the river banks were removed to make way for the increased water flows, caused by the construction of the Snowy Mountains hydroelectricity and irrigation scheme. I was once given a joey kangaroo after his mother had been killed by a pack of dogs. He was still a baby but covered with fur, and transitioning from living in his mother's pouch and having her milk to eating grass. The mother had thrown him from the pouch as she tried to escape the dogs. I kept him in a hessian pouch-like bag next to the coke-fired, hot-water heater to keep him warm, and fed him a recipe of cow's milk obtained from the Taronga Park Zoo. The zoo staff had told me to return the joey to his mother or he would not survive. Despite my best efforts, the baby did not thrive and eventually succumbed to pneumonia during the winter. Breastmilk protects infants from infection, and without the antibodies from his mother's milk, like human babies, the young joey could not fight off the infection.

My father was opposed to me having a university education. He believed a woman did not need to be educated, as she would marry and be supported by her husband. This was a paradox, because without Mum's accounting expertise and energy, he would never have managed to run the family business. In the sixties, without a scholarship or other financial means, nursing or teaching were the only feasible options for country girls who wanted a career. The kindness of the nurses during my illness and the many nurses within my family pushed me towards nursing.

Living in the Philippines

In Year 11, I won a Rotary scholarship to live in the Philippines for a year. Throughout 1970, I lived with eight different Rotary families in Mindanao, a province in the southern Philippines. Upon arrival, my first foster father told me to be careful, saying life was as cheap as a chicken in Cotabato City. He told me there was great inequity in the country, and some people were desperate. My role as a Rotary student was to be an ambassador for the Corryong Rotary club and fit in. I was not to become involved in politics. I attended Notre Dame

University throughout the year, while studying Tagalog and Filipino history, and learning to play the guitar and mah-jong.

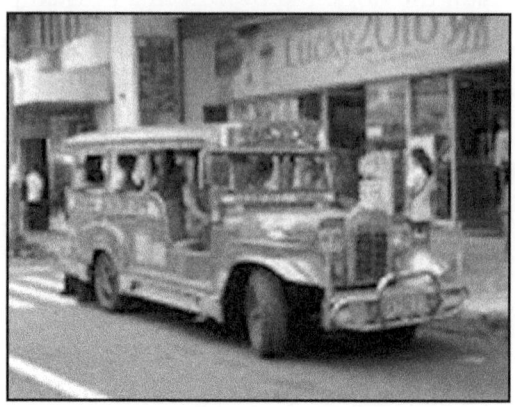

Jeepney, local public transport in Mindanao, 1970

My foster sisters encouraged me to join a sorority, which was really a girls' club for having fun with sister members. Some of the sisters were political activists. I had great freedom, made many friends among the Catholic and Muslim communities, and was able to get about using jeepneys. Many students opposed the excesses of President Ferdinand Marcos and his wife, Imelda. While Marcos and his government labelled student activists 'communists', the activists called him an 'American puppet'. Rumours abounded of students going missing, with some reports saying they were being thrown into the sea from government helicopters.

Having had an idyllic childhood growing up in the countryside, surrounded by a loving family and plenty of food on the table, I had found the poverty and inequity in Mindanao a great shock. A large proportion of the predominantly Catholic country was living in appalling poverty, while elections were rigged with bribery and coercion. I was fascinated when my family took me to a polling booth during a council election. Uniformed police and soldiers with guns watched on as cash was handed to voters. Corruption of politicians had allowed multinational companies to come to Mindanao and exploit the natural materials, with little recompense to the locals. Land clearing and logging had resulted in mudslides, death and destruction. The provinces' resources were being looted. In 1972, martial law was declared.

I returned home at the end of 1970 in time for Christmas, and became the butt of racism and teasing, due to the very strong Filipino accent I had acquired. I had come to love my Filipino families and friends and was appalled by the racist taunts. I had also come to doubt the Australian Government's reason for entering the Vietnam War. While in the Philippines, I discovered that 'the yellow peril' was actually a description of poor people who wanted a decent life, and communism was an ideology promising a fairer share.

After a year away, my parents were challenged by their independent and changed daughter. I was bored with the idea of returning to school and dreaded the thought of being under the control of my parents for another year. I knew they would expect me to work long hours in the family business for pocket money. I wanted to get on with my life, so in April 1971 I accepted a place in the earliest possible intake of nursing students at The Royal Melbourne Hospital.

Training to be a nurse

It was an exciting time to be in Melbourne as the baby boomers were coming of age. Germaine Greer, a Melbourne-born writer, had published *The Female Eunuch* in 1970. Her thesis became an international bestseller and a pivotal text within the feminist movement. Greer believed that the traditional suburban family repressed women sexually and challenged us all to question the power of traditional authority figures, such as priests, doctors and police.

In 1972, Australia's twenty-first prime minister, Gough Whitlam, was voted into office, ending Australia's involvement in the Vietnam War. The conservative Australian Liberal Government had believed the capitalist system was under threat from communism, and Australia was actively involved in the Vietnam War between 1965 and 1972. Like the Americans, the conservatives believed in the 'domino theory', which likened non-communist states and nearby communist states to falling dominos and feared the spread of communism throughout the world. During Australia's involvement in the war, 15,300 20-year-old Australian boys were conscripted by birth dates into the Australian Army. More than 200 died in Vietnam, and at least 1200 were wounded on active duty. Many boys returned home with post-traumatic stress-related injuries.

I trained as a general nurse at the Royal Melbourne from 1971 to 1974. During the first year, I lived in the nurses' home and enjoyed the camaraderie and support of most of the 64 other young women who began in the preliminary training school (PTS). The first six weeks were spent living in Toorak, in the leafy eastern suburbs in a stately home called 'Trawalla'. We were herded onto the hospital bus early weekday mornings in starched uniforms and caps and driven to Parkville, a suburb that housed the hospital and The University of Melbourne.

In PTS, we learned the fundamentals of caring for the sick. We were expected to study different medical and surgical subjects, and take part in practical sessions that would equip us for entering the wards to work as junior nurses. Our training included making different types of beds to ensure patient comfort, including a standard hospital bed with crisp white linen, an operation bed with folded sheet and blanket bed pack, and divided linen beds for orthopaedic patients to allow broken limbs to be elevated discreetly. All were practised until we were able to perfect hospital corners. How to give a bed bath, clean false teeth and deliver a bedpan were all part of the practical education. The changing of the sputum mug was particularly gross.

During the six weeks, we formed enduring friendship groups and spent the evenings talking and laughing about what we had learned. At Trawalla, we were a short walk to coffee shops and cinemas or, for the more adventurous, trams into the city. In the sixth week of the preliminary training school we took exams. Those who succeeded were given annual leave for a week, while those who failed were asked to leave. Following PTS, we were moved onsite to the hospital grounds and housed in the multi-storeyed redbrick nurses' home, a short walk from the hospital wards where we were rostered to work.

My first ward was 6 North, consisting of an open renal ward housing 16 men separated by curtains, and shared four-, two- and one-bed rooms along a corridor, mainly housing women. Single rooms were kept for private patients, those with infections or patients most in need, such as those who were dying. Halfway along the corridor was the nurses' station with views into the wards, and a panel with patient bed numbers that lit up when the call bell was pressed.

On each level of the nine-storeyed building, lifts carried the users of the hospital to a central point where, at each compass point, there was a ward. During the day, a junior nurse, under the supervision of a senior second- or third-year nurse (shown by the number of red stripes on their cap), was responsible for the care of half of the patients each end of the 30-bed wards. A registered nurse was in charge of the entire ward and the student nurses.

The morning shift consisted of making each patient's bed and orchestrating patient hygiene. This meant assisting patients with a bath, showering or a bed bath, teeth cleaning and two-hourly pressure care rounds for the bedridden, which could involve lifting heavy, immobile patients. We helped feed those patients who needed feeding after the charge nurse had served up meals from hot mobile food trolleys, which were delivered to the wards each mealtime. Electric stainless-steel trolleys were plugged in, and the required diets were dished up from large steel tubs. Ensuring that each patient was ready for the meal, by being sat up with a linen serviette in place, was the job of the junior and senior nurses.

In the renal ward, most patients were on fluid balance charts, and it was the junior nurse's role on morning shifts to make sure that a large portion of fluid intake was delivered before the shift's end. The job was arduous, as many patients did not want to drink, while patients on restricted fluids were thirsty and wanted more. If a patient had not drunk their quota by the shift's end, we would be chastised and made to remain behind until they did.

On every fourth week, on Saturdays, we were required to finish two hours earlier at 1:30 pm so we could work a split shift on Sunday. This shortened Saturday shift was particularly galling, as most of the work was required to be done before we went off. Pushing fluids on unwilling patients was particularly difficult. The next day, Sunday, we were rostered to work from 7:00 am until 1:30 pm. We had to get through the normal eight hours work in six hours and return to the ward at 5:00 pm, covering the tea break and getting on with the evening workload. We finished at 9:00 pm instead of 11:00 pm, but it was rare to get off shortened shifts on time, and we would go home exhausted.

The ward rounds by the doctors were anticipated with high expectations. At a regular time on weekday mornings, after the ward had been readied, a suited gentleman surrounded by registrars and junior doctors in long white coats would enter the ward, with medical students in short white coats and the white-veiled charge nurse. Our charge nurse was a blonde beauty, always immaculate in her uniform and gossiped about, as it was speculated she was in love with the consultant doctor. A patient's bed was surrounded by the entourage. One by one all the patients were examined, while their medical conditions were discussed with the students and junior doctors, who learned from the consultation. The charge nurse took notes, which she later disseminated to the nurses, who altered the care as required.

At meal breaks, we were served hearty meals in the hospital dining room at tables designated according to rank in the hospital hierarchy. There was little intermingling. Smoking was still permitted in the dining room; smoke permeated throughout and cigarettes could be obtained at cafeteria vending machines.

Throughout the three-year training program, we had regular study blocks and exams. However, I recall no breastfeeding education during the course. A short walk down Flemington Road from the Royal Melbourne was The Royal Children's Hospital (RCH); nurses from the children's hospital were sent to the Royal Melbourne to experience adult nursing and vice versa. In 1972, over Christmas and New Year, I undertook children's nursing at the RCH, with my first placement in the neonatal intensive care unit for babies with the sorts of abnormalities we do not see today due to ultrasound. Most babies were kept in incubators and fed by tube. Although a very junior nurse, I found the lack of parental involvement odd and did not know the difference between expressed breastmilk and commercial baby milk. The neonatal nursery appeared to me more like a scientific laboratory and the little babies inside the incubators, specimens on display.

In my second year I was required to repeat the dietetics (the study of food and nutrition to optimise health) exam and just passed the supplementary exam, despite sleeping in and arriving late. We had thought the dietetics exam was a joke, as the quality of teaching was poor and the content inadequate, so we had not taken it seriously. But if I had failed again, I would have been asked to leave. Neither breastfeeding nor breastmilk was discussed.

What I remember of my nursing course was three years of hard shift work, study and lectures in a hierarchical, male-dominated establishment, where mainly young women were exploited as cheap labour, while on the good side obtaining a qualification in nursing that was recognised worldwide. We were supervised by the female enforcers, that is, women who belong to the status quo, who were supporting a patriarchal system and did the caring work relied upon by the hospital and community for a small wage, accommodation, food and health care. However, unlike nursing students of today, we were not saddled with debt and were work ready when our course was complete. If we chose to become a midwife, we were expected to undertake another year of training at a maternity hospital.

My birthing experience

I was 22 years old when my first baby was born in 1975. Like most first-time parents, my partner Jim and I were excited but full of trepidation. Having been born following the Second World War, we were part of the emerging baby boomers.

French obstetrician Frederick Leboyer had published *Birth without Violence* in 1974, a book which focused on the needs of the infant. He advocated for gentle birthing in a quiet and dimly lit delivery room to prevent sensory overload, while keeping the mother close rather than taking the baby to a nursery. We shopped around Melbourne looking for a birthing hospital that practised the Leboyer method. None did.

At the first visit to the public maternity outpatients close to my home in Fitzroy I waited – stripped of my clothing and in a cold white hospital gown – to see the doctor. After the vaginal examination confirming the pregnancy, I left the hospital crying. Rather than care for my pregnancy, the elderly male had chastised me as an unmarried mother. He then intimated that I would be unfit to raise a child and should go back to the hospital where I worked and have something done. I worked at The Queen Victoria Hospital for Women and Children, but preferred to birth elsewhere to keep my private and professional life separate. Without asking about my social situation, the doctor had asserted his religious and conservative bigotry in his role as a health professional and had presumed that not being married would make me unfit to be a mother.

Eventually, after much discussion with friends and colleagues, and a lack of satisfactory options, we chose to be cared for privately by a respected female obstetrician from the Queen Vic. Jim accompanied me to the first antenatal appointment, and the doctor began the consultation by examining our social situation. When she learned we were happy and excited about our impending baby, she listened to our birth plan and tried to accommodate our wishes, agreeing that Jim could be with me during the labour and birth, which was unusual at that time.

When I went into labour, I was fit and well and in a great place mentally. We had recently returned from a camping holiday in Queensland, where we had swum every day in the waves of the warm tropical waters, eaten the locally grown fruits and foods sold along the roadsides, and made love. I birthed an almost 4-kilogram, perfect baby girl, after labouring mostly alone. I had arrived by taxi at Jessie McPherson, the private wing of the Queen Vic having contractions every five minutes. Sophie, Jim's sister, accompanied me, as Jim was on night shift. I was led to the delivery room and Sophie was told by the midwife to go home. I was assessed and then left alone in the dark. Lying on the bed, I remembered the breathing strategies from the antenatal classes, as the contractions become stronger and closer together.

When the contractions were almost on top of one another and allowing little rest, I asked where Jim was. I also requested some pain relief, as the pain had become intolerable. I was given pethidine. Not long after the injection, I felt the pressure of the infant's head on my bowel and asked for a bedpan. Trying to balance on the pan in the bed alone, as the nurse had told me not to get out of bed was mad, as my head was spinning from the pethidine. I felt the membranes 'pop' and the waters around the baby's head gush into the pan. I told the midwife that the membranes had broken, and she replied, 'Don't be silly, dear'.

Where was Jim? And why wasn't he here to advocate for me as we'd planned? Soon after the pan was taken away, there was a flurry of activity and the lights were turned on. A covered trolley was wheeled into the room. The doctor arrived and asked where Jim was. Jim later told me he had been called shortly before the birth and jumped onto his push bike to race into the city. It was morning peak hour. He arrived just as the baby was born and took my hand, which he held until we heard the baby cry. It seemed like an eternity. She required considerable resuscitation following delivery, which included oxygen, assisted breathing with a bag, and mask and medications to reverse the effects of the pethidine. We were told the cord was around the baby's neck.

After becoming a midwife, I realised many babies were born with the cord around the neck and lack of monitoring during labour had contributed to the midwife giving pethidine too close to the birth. Had I been given nitrous and oxygen to breathe or perhaps a kind word and some encouragement, the pethidine might not have been necessary. Drugged and exhausted, I slept all day. The baby had been born at 10:01 am, and I did not wake until Jim returned during visiting hours later that evening. I had not breastfed following the birth, and the baby had been taken to the nursery and cared for there during the crucial initial breastfeeding and bonding period.

At that time at Jessie McPherson, visitors were restricted to the woman's partner or the infant's grandparents for the first three days. Jim came as often as work allowed, but my family did not. Dad was furious that we had not married and made all sorts of threats to force our hand, while Mum was the meat in the sandwich. She called me frequently on the telephone, making sure I had everything I needed. But as the midwives were disapproving of personal calls, we did not speak for long. Mum could not come to Melbourne to visit, as she was essential to the everyday needs of the hotel, six hours' drive from Melbourne. She was an amazing woman who worked from seven in the morning until ten at night, six days a week.

Keeping babies in the nursery was standard care in maternity hospitals when my first baby was born. The rationale was that if babies were kept separate from their mothers it would prevent infection. In fact, the opposite is true. The infant's bacteria is colonised from the mother when placed skin-to-skin rather than from the nursery and hospital staff. Babies were often fed breast-milk substitutes in the nursery between feeds, and occasionally the wrong baby was taken to the wrong mother. Babies were only brought to their mother's bedside every four hours for feeding. They could be viewed through a glass nursery window at other times.

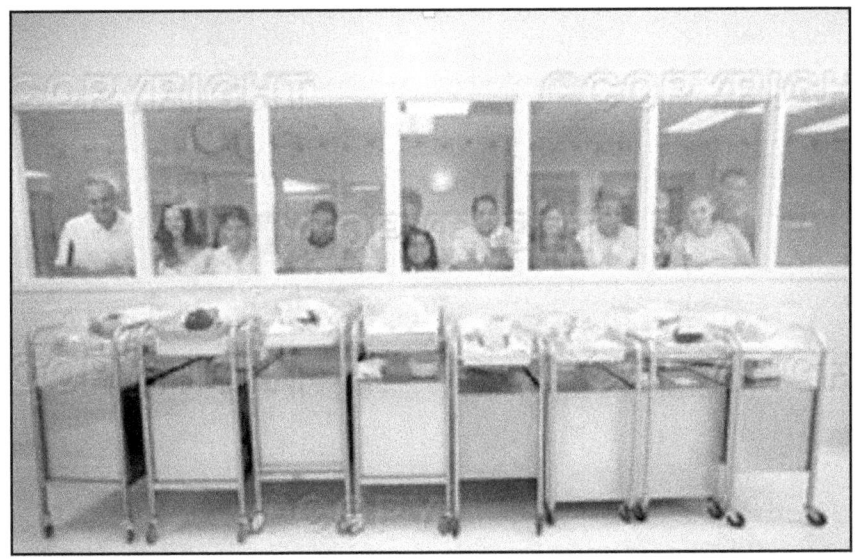

Parents viewing infants at visiting hours in a hospital nursery, 1975. Getty Images

A particular routine was followed during my time in hospital. In the first 24 hours, my baby was permitted to remain on the breast for three minutes each side. On the second day, the time at the breast was increased to five minutes, and on the third day following birth, seven minutes. Looking back as a lactation consultant, this seems ludicrous. During the second 24-hour period post birth, it is normal infant behaviour to cluster feed to stimulate breastmilk production. In a normal, healthy-term baby, small frequent feeds of colostrum are required to satisfy a baby, as the infant's tummy is small and the baby has extra brown fat to sustain the transition from the placenta to full breastfeeding.

I awoke during the night three days after the birth, feeling my breasts would explode, and went to the nursery needing to feed. Rather than wake me, the nursery staff had bottle-fed my baby with something other than my milk, and I was told to use the electric pump and express to relieve the engorgement. There was only one midwife throughout my entire hospital stay who sat with me and gave me information about positioning and attachment and helped me to breastfeed. I remained in hospital for the required 10 days, feeling alone and isolated. There was a strong conservatism in hospitals in the early 1970s that reflected the ideas of the past. As a single mother, I think many of the staff thought I had the plague and allowed their bigotry to impact my care. These were the same people who pressured single mothers to give up their infants.

I had entered hospital an excited and confident young mother wanting to breastfeed. Towards the end of the 10-day hospital stay, my obstetrician prescribed antidepressants, as the midwives said I appeared unhappy. I threw them onto the garden under the window beside my bed rather than argue.

Learning to parent

My baby was born on 6 November 1975. Prime Minister Gough Whitlam was sacked during my hospital stay. I watched the protestors from the Swanston Street window as they marched through the city, and remember thinking that he may have stopped the Vietnam War but things needed to improve for women.

After leaving hospital, I returned to Jim's parents' home with the baby because he was still working at night. Like many mothers-in-law before her, Jim's mother did not make my life easy, and we quickly moved out into a shared house in a leafy eastern suburb with Jim's sister, Genevieve, her husband, Des, and another couple. It was wonderful sharing the house with people who loved our daughter and were prepared to help. My brother-in-law was a baby whisperer. In the evening when I was tired and she was crying, he would pick up the baby and take her walking and return her to me contentedly asleep on his shoulder. Genevieve was an excellent cook, and she would make beautiful meals for us all.

I remained at home enjoying the time with my baby until Jim completed his term at the hospital. He became a house husband, while I returned to work in the operating room of a private hospital close to home. Jim bottle-fed commercial baby milk when I was working and I breastfed when at home. Jim loved that time sharing our baby's care with his sister and Des, who had no children of their own. Although I did feel regret leaving the baby, I also enjoyed being the breadwinner and the stimulation of the work and my colleagues.

Due to Christmas and New Year, the six-week postnatal doctor's appointment was delayed. I did not know it at the time, but I was already pregnant. Jim and I thought breastfeeding was a contraceptive and I did not understand that I needed to express regularly when I recommenced work. I should have been expressing when Jim was bottle-feeding. We did not realise that, if the breastfeeding hormones dropped due to a lack of frequent emptying of the breasts, breastmilk supply would fall, and ovulation may occur. Although I was a trained registered nurse from the Royal Melbourne and Royal Children's hospitals, and had attended childbirth and breastfeeding classes prior to having a baby, I was poorly informed. I did not know that, to increase breastmilk supply to meet the growing baby's needs, I needed to feed more often. I thought if I rested my breasts and gave a bottle, I would have more milk next time. In the nursery after I breastfed, they topped up the babies with bottled milk, which I believed was required.

Australian Breastfeeding Association

Amy Brown, a researcher from the United Kingdom, found many women carry their lack of achieving breastfeeding success as a grief throughout their life (Brown, 2018). On a personal level, I would say this is true.

In the 1960s, Mary Paton and a group of five other mothers from Melbourne recognised the lack of professional support for breastfeeding women and had set up the Nursing Mothers' Association. I was sad that I had not breastfed for a longer period and joined the Association in 1976 in the hope that I would do better with my second baby. Receiving their regular newsletter supported and connected me with other breastfeeding mothers.

The Nursing Mother's Association became the Australian Breastfeeding Association (ABA) in 2001 and currently has 350,000 members throughout Australia. ABA is responsible for much of the evidence-based breastfeeding research and education supplied to health professionals and breastfeeding women. The ABA recognised that health professionals lacked breastfeeding expertise and that there was a great need in the community for breastfeeding help.

The second labour

The birth of our second daughter changed our lives and inadvertently caused us to leave Australia. Jessica was born at the Mansfield Hospital where we had moved after our first daughter was born. I had been happy and well throughout the pregnancy, enjoying my time at home in the small country town. Close to the due date and late in the afternoon, I attended the obstetrician's rooms, with our daughter in the stroller as she was not yet walking, for a regular antenatal appointment. The obstetrician took my blood pressure and asked me to lie on the couch, where she checked the baby's growth

Patriarchy, Misogyny and Breastfeeding

by feeling my abdomen and listened to the baby's heartbeat with a Pinard's stethoscope. A Pinard's stethoscope is a hollow horn, often made of wood or metal, about 20 centimetres long and used for amplifying sound. The obstetrician told me I was in labour. I laughed, responding that I had been having irregular contractions on and off for nearly two months. She then said my baby had foetal distress and I needed to go to the hospital immediately.

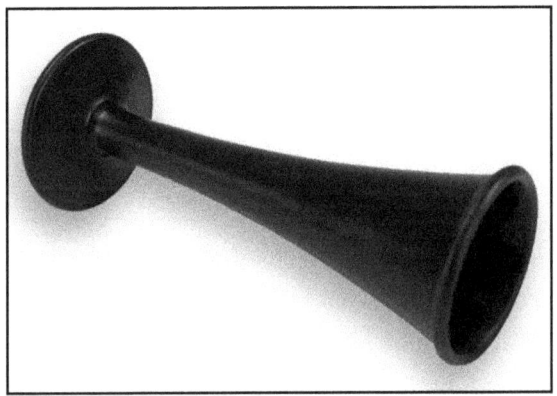

Pinard's stethoscope used for listening to a baby's heartbeat in utero

To say I was surprised was an understatement. I felt great, and I was a perfectly fit non-smoking, healthy young woman. As a result of local gossip, I did not completely trust the doctor and told her I wanted to speak with Jim. I should have gone home and telephoned him. But it was before mobile phones, and as he was on duty at the hospital, I put our daughter in the stroller and walked there to find him. I was not prepared for the midwife and another staff member waiting for me at the reception desk when we arrived.

They did not get Jim as I requested and took my daughter forcefully from my arms, leading me to the labour ward with her cries ringing in my ears. Without consent or any discussion, I was administered pethidine and Phenergan. In those days, I barely took a Panadol, so these drugs knocked me out. I did ask the staff before they did anything to wait until I could speak with Jim, but I was ignored. While I was drowsy and under the influence of the drugs and, again, without my consent, my legs were placed in stirrups and the doctor performed a vaginal examination and ruptured the membranes around the baby.

Jim had been delayed as he was organising a babysitter. When he finally arrived, I was in a drugged sleep. Later, he told me when he asked the obstetrician the reason for the induction that she had said it was an emergency situation due to foetal distress. When she said this he had looked at the midwife, who had blushed. She, like the obstetrician, was a colleague. He asked the midwife the baby's heart rate and she replied it was normal. She also told him the waters around the baby had been clear, which is most unusual with foetal distress.

Jim had overestimated the obstetrician. He had mistakenly thought she would be mindful of our wishes and expectations, as they were colleagues. We had been told she was a nine-to-five deliverer by friends in the town, but we were naive. The doctor wanted to go away for the weekend, as she had an important meeting in Melbourne. After the induction she told Jim that, if he was not happy with her care, she could arrange for an ambulance to transfer me to Wangaratta or Melbourne. He replied that we would have taken that option if it had been offered prior to rupturing the membranes. But because of the risk of infection once the membranes had been ruptured, there was not much we could do.

At around 2:00 am I was asleep and not contracting. Jim woke me to tell me not to sign anything. He whispered that the obstetrician was getting tired and organising the operating theatre for a caesarean section. Perhaps it was the adrenalin, but very soon after I started to contract and Jessica was born. I remained in the quiet country hospital for five days, resting and getting to know my newborn while establishing breastfeeding. Genevieve and Des collected our eldest child and cared for her in Melbourne while I was in hospital. The midwives let me do my own thing. I kept Jessie at the bedside or in bed with me, feeding her whenever she wanted and only returning her to the nursery when I slept. The midwives were kind and made time to help me and the few other women in the postnatal ward. When I left hospital, I was exclusively breastfeeding and did so for six months, when we introduced family foods. I continued to breastfeed for more than two years.

Jim resigned from the general practice the morning following Jessie's birth. He was furious. He said he could no longer work there, saying the doctor had behaved in an unethical manner. She was later named in the Victorian Parliament as the obstetrician with the greatest number of inductions in the state. We returned to Melbourne with two young infants, unemployed. Jim was unsure of his future. He had disliked not following through with the patients' care after diagnosing their issues and getting to know them. For anything serious, they needed to be referred to the big city or base hospitals.

A friend from his residency days had recently returned from two years on the island of Manus in Papua New Guinea (PNG) and suggested we give PNG a try. He told us not to agree to work in any sole position and gave us the direct line to a recruitment officer known to process applicants quickly. Within days, we boarded the Bird of Paradise at Tullamarine and left Australia, having signed a two-year contract.

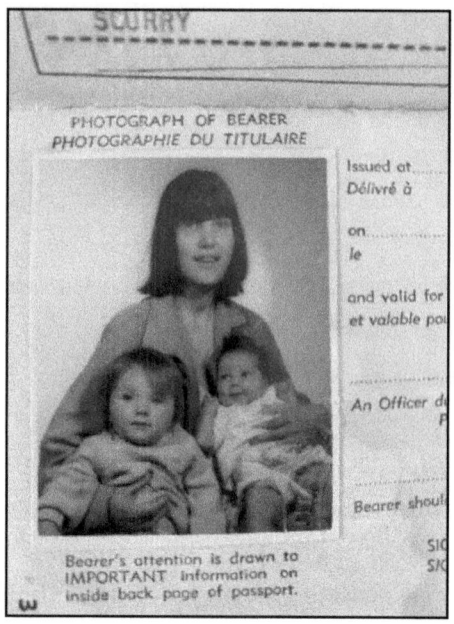

Passport to Papua New Guinea with two very young daughters, 1976

Life in Papua New Guinea

We lived in Kimbe, PNG and I worked in the local hospital five mornings a week as a qualified general nurse. I was in awe of the Melanesian midwives, who I watched fascinated from the general wards as mothers laboured. The labouring women swayed to and fro as their labour progressed, bending to the rhythms of the contractions. The women wandered on the hospital lawns accompanied by other women, talking and laughing and eating the foods they liked, watched over by the midwives who were close at hand to assist when required. The midwives were highly skilled and could deliver most births. There were few doctors in the provinces, and the midwives were able to use a ventouse suction cap, when necessary, as it was considered safer than forceps. Kimbe was situated between the sea and a mountain range, with emergency flights only possible during the day. Women requiring a caesarean section or specialist services were flown out prior to the due date of birth.

I was sorry I had not been cared for by midwives when my daughters were born. I know the arguments, but birth and breastfeeding could be done so much better in Australia if consumers had a greater input into the type of care offered and there were no vested interests. Travelling to PNG and being exposed to its culture gave us the opportunity to look at birth with new eyes. 'It takes a village to raise a child' took on new meaning. Unlike the nuclear families of today, women in the village shared their lives with aunties, grandmothers, and other mothers and girls, and they also shared childcare. If the mother was ill or had died, they shared breastfeeding. When the women needed to work in the gardens, the baby was placed in a *bilum* (string bag) on the mother's back. The babies appeared to cry less than my girls, as they were rocked with the constant movement and were in close contact with their mother. At night, they slept on a mat beside their mother on the floor and fed when hungry, as they were within easy access of the breast. If babies were hospitalised, the mothers slept with them in the hospital, breastfeeding and providing care.

My babies slept in their own beds as I was taught to have them do by my mother and grandmother. I got little rest, as they cried often, and I was constantly woken up and trying to settle them. At that time in Australia, *Toddler Taming*, a book by Christopher Green, promoted controlled crying and was widely shared among parents. I could not let Jessie cry it out, as we lived in a compound in Kimbe with louvre windows close to our neighbours. So I moved Jessica into our bed to prevent the neighbours being disturbed. Often it was all four of us in the bed or Jim moving into another bed so we could rest. It seemed such a natural thing to do and bizarre that I had not rejected the cruelty of leaving my babies alone in the dark back in Australia. I can clearly remember being terrified of the dark as a child and imagining crocodiles under the bed. For many years, my brother and I shared a room because he, too, was afraid and had nightmares.

In PNG, I saw babies die from lack of breastfeeding due to commercial baby milk manufacturers marketing their product to an uneducated population. I was encouraged by Stephen Oppenheimer, a paediatrician working in PNG for WHO, to breastfeed my daughter wherever and whenever she was hungry. Steve was implementing the *Susu Bilong Mama* (breastfeeding) public health campaign. He explained that in PNG feeding commercial baby milk was a status symbol for Melanesian women and he wanted me to demonstrate that some white women also breastfeed.

Life decisions

When we returned to Australia in 1980, the wonderful work of the PNG midwives was directly responsible for my decision to study midwifery and lactation. I wanted to try and improve the lives of birthing and breastfeeding women and their families.

I have spent most of my working life juggling family and paid work with women and babies in Australia and overseas. In 2021, I undertook a Masters of Midwifery research project looking at the impact of the postnatal ward environment on breastfeeding.

I have been happily married to Jim for over 45 years and have five grown-up children and seven grandchildren. I have helped my daughters and our sons' partners breastfeed all of their babies according to WHO recommendations. Over many years, I have helped a large number of women achieve their breastfeeding goals. In writing down the knowledge I have gained, my aim is to inform the breastfeeding debate and demonstrate how patriarchy and misogyny, as well as colonisation and capitalism, have impacted the ability of Australian women to mother.

2

Breastfeeding as a Human Rights Issue

Following the devastation of the First and Second World Wars and the deaths of millions, Australia became a signatory to the 1948 United Nations General Assembly Universal Declaration of Human Rights, which stated: 'We the peoples of the United Nations are determined to save succeeding generations from the scourge of war, which twice in our lifetime has brought untold sorrow to mankind' (United Nations, 1948). In describing human rights in 1958, Eleanor Roosevelt who had chaired the Human Rights Commission said:

> Where do Human Rights begin? In small places, close to home – so close and so small that they cannot be seen on any maps of the world. Yet they are the world of the individual person; the neighbourhood he lives in; the school or college he attends; the factory, farm or office where he works. Such are the places where every man, woman, and child seek equal justice, equal opportunity, equal dignity without discrimination. Unless these rights have meaning there, they have little meaning anywhere. Without concerted citizen action to uphold them close to home, we shall look in vain for progress in the larger world.

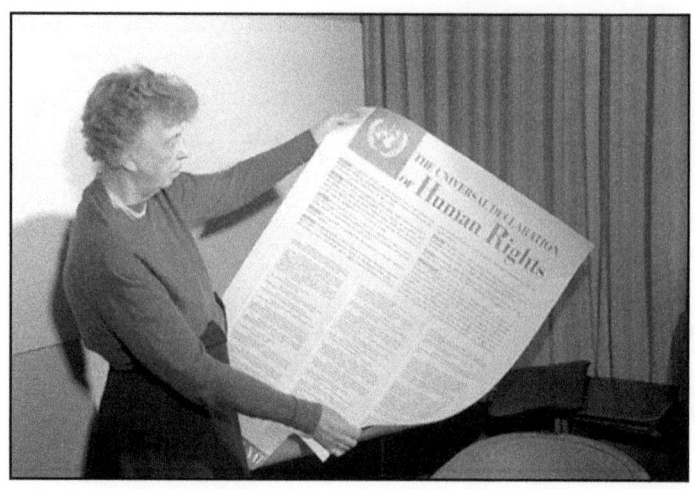

Eleanor Roosevelt and the Human Rights Charter, 1948. UN photo.

Human rights agreements were adopted to protect the rights of all humans, no matter their age, sex, race, colour, religion, or economic or social background, and to prevent future conflict. The Convention on the Elimination of all Forms of Discrimination against Women adopted in 1979 by the United Nations General Assembly states, 'Discrimination against women violates the principles of equality of rights and respect for human dignity, and is an obstacle to the participation of women on equal terms with men. Discriminatory practices against women hamper the growth of society and families and make it more difficult the reach the full development of the potentialities of women in the service of their countries and of humanity' (United Nations General Assembly, 1979). The Convention's Article 5 states:

> Parties shall take all appropriate measures:
>
> To modify the social and cultural patterns of conduct of men and women, with a view to achieving the elimination of prejudices and customary and all other practices which are based on the idea of the

inferiority or the superiority of either of the sexes or on stereotyped roles for men and women;

To ensure that family education includes a proper understanding of maternity as a social function and the recognition of the common responsibility of men and women in the upbringing and development of their children, it being understood that the interest of the children is the primordial consideration in all cases.

The Convention on the Rights of the Child, adopted in 1989, recognises the child's inherent right to life, survival and development, including a state of complete physical, mental and social wellbeing. Breastfeeding is fundamental to optimum infant nutrition.

A fundamental human right

Australia has no bill of rights. However, as a signatory to the United Nations General Assembly Universal Declaration of Human Rights, Australia has a responsibility to uphold them, and any attempt to justify discrimination against women is unacceptable.

WHO recommends breastfeeding by the infant's mother as the first option of choice. If the baby cannot breastfeed for any reason, WHO recommends the baby be fed the mother's own expressed breastmilk. If this is not possible, donor milk from another human mother is the next best alternative, for example the breastmilk of a family member or friend, or donor milk obtained from a human milk bank. The majority of commercial baby milk is obtained from cows and not designed for human infants, so should be viewed as an emergency substitute food.

During the twentieth century, arguably because of high infant and maternal mortality rates, governments around the world encouraged birthing within the hospital setting. The hospital setting medicalised birth and took the focus off mothering. Women generally do not want to leave their communities to birth in a large centralised city hospital. In my health district, when a local maternity facility was to be closed, the community protested and applied political pressure to keep the facility open. While the obstetric service was closed and replaced by a less expensive model, the care of well women within the community was retained and continues to support one-on-one midwifery-led birthing at home and in a birthing centre. Most women want their partner or family members to support them when having a baby, as birth, like death, is a normal life event.

Healthy women and children are the foundation stones of a healthy society. Copious research studies have demonstrated that women have been dissatisfied with postnatal care within hospitals and the community for decades, and breastfeeding statistics in Australia demonstrate there is a problem. Mothers and children are a valuable resource, and well-targeted interventions can provide healthy children to produce the nation's wealth.

In Australia, because of historical gender inequity, half of the nation's population has been denied power and excluded from decision-making. Women given the responsibility of home-making and raising children have little say in the decisions that impact them, while many women in positions of power do not understand the plight of new mothers and do not have the knowledge to advocate for them. When tax dollars are spent, the loyalties of politicians will be swayed by the parties' financial backers, and precious health dollars may be directed away from vulnerable women and children.

In 2010, I was an observer at the Baby-Friendly Hospital Initiative (BFHI) country coordinators meeting of industrialised nations in Florence, Italy. The UNICEF Innocenti Research Centre, where the meeting was held, had been an orphanage. Predominantly female babies were housed within the building in the former Hospital of the Innocents. Within the historic building built in 1419, is a museum that tells the story of the orphans who resided there. The mortality rate was 100 per cent for babies not returned to their mothers or a wet nurse.

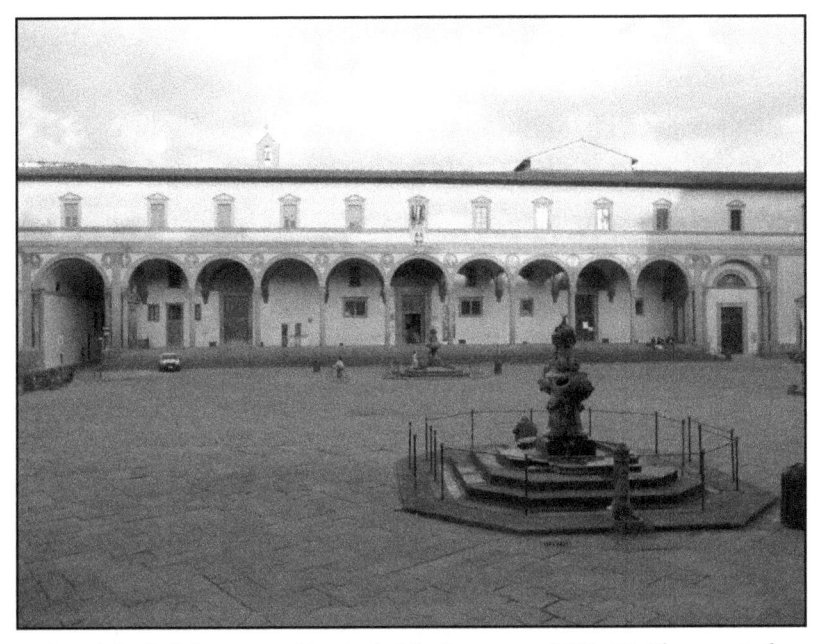

Ospedale degli Innocenti, Hospital of the Innocents, 1419–51, Florence, Italy

As a founding member of the United Nations, Australia has a political imperative to uphold the targets of the Sustainable Development Goals (SDGs), which were adopted by the United Nations in 2015. The 17 SDGs are designed to balance social, economic and environmental sustainability, with the aim of ending poverty, hunger, AIDS, and discrimination against women and girls. Maternal, infant and young child nutrition targets for 2030 include increasing the rate of exclusive breastfeeding in the first six months up to at least 50 per cent of all infants (WHO, 2014). The World Health Assembly maternal, infant and young child nutritional targets to be achieved by 2030 are listed in Figure 2.1.

Figure 2.1: Six Global Infant Nutrition Targets

1. Achieve a 40 per cent reduction in the number of children under 5 who are stunted.
2. Achieve a 50 per cent reduction of anaemia in women of reproductive age.
3. Achieve a 30 per cent reduction in low birth weight.
4. Ensure that there is no increase in childhood overweight.
5. Increase the rate of exclusive breastfeeding in the first six months up to at least 50 per cent.
6. Reduce and maintain childhood wasting to less than 5 per cent (WHO, 2014).

Marketing breastmilk substitutes

WHO and UNICEF have advocated for many years that infants be breastfed by their mothers. In 1974, the 27th World Health Assembly, recognising the general decline in breastfeeding and the impact of the production, marketing and advertising of manufactured breastmilk substitutes on breastfeeding families, encouraged member states to implement a minimal acceptable standard for marketing substitute baby milk as a way to improve the health and nutrition of infants and young children.

In 1981, the 33rd World Health Assembly adopted the WHO Code as a minimum acceptable requirement for the marketing breastmilk substitutes, with the aim of protecting and promoting breastfeeding and ensuring that marketing of breastmilk substitutes, feeding bottles and teats is done appropriately. The code applies to both companies and governments.

In 2007, a federal parliamentary inquiry into breastfeeding in Australia recognised that the Manufacturers and Importers Agreement (MAIF), which is a voluntary, self-regulatory code of conduct operated by members of the Infant Nutrition Council, was inadequate and recommended that Australia adopt the WHO code. Recommendation 22 encourages 'the Department of Health and Ageing [to] adopt the World Health Organization's International Code of Marketing of Breast-Milk Substitutes and subsequent World Health Assembly resolutions'.

The inquiry identified that, 'The aggressive marketing of breastmilk substitutes creates a major barrier to breastfeeding. Following the adoption of the International Code of Marketing of Breast-Milk Substitutes in 1981, governments have been called upon repeatedly by the World Health Assembly to give effect to the provisions in the Code through national legislation' (Commonwealth of Australia, 2007).

The recommendation was not implemented, and Australia continues to market non-human baby milk products for human babies, despite copious evidence that demonstrates that breastmilk is optimum and that most women can breastfeed if given timely, accurate support. The WHO Code for Marketing Breastmilk Substitutes in Australia has no legal status and the MAIF agreement does not regulate supermarket or chemist sales of commercial baby milk, so continues to operate as an ineffective tool. There are many examples of breaches of marketing practices by manufacturers of commercial baby milk. Due to the many differing silos and priorities within health, hospital managers in maternity within BFHI-accredited facilities need to remain vigilant. Education events sponsored by commercial baby milk manufacturers may impact what some health professionals tell parents and the hard-earned rigorous processes required to maintain BFHI accreditation status.

Figure 2.2: National Legal Status of WHO Code for Marketing Breastmilk Substitutes, 2020. Source: WHO, 2020

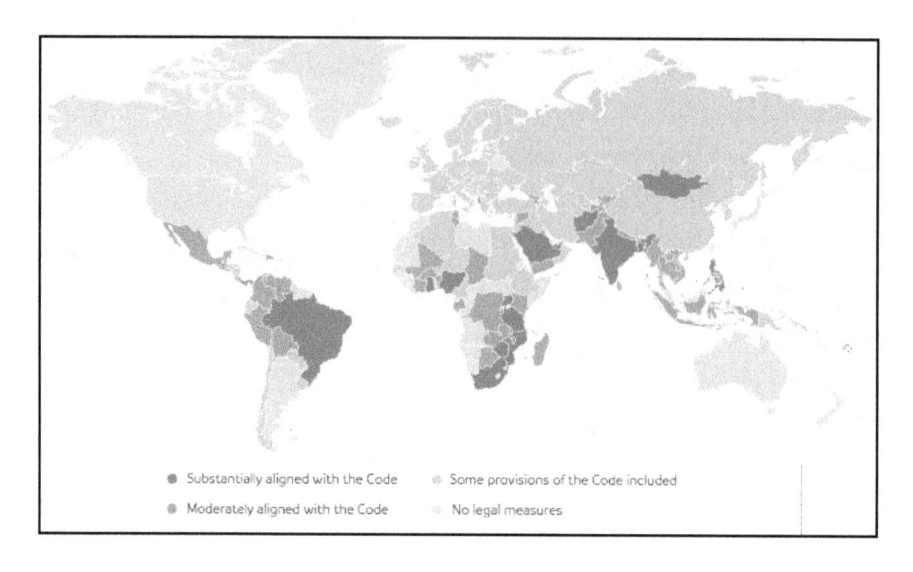

[Map of the world showing national legal status, with legend: Substantially aligned with the Code; Some provisions of the Code included; Moderately aligned with the Code; No legal measures]

In 2016, *The Lancet* stated, 'The marketing of breast-milk substitutes negatively affects breastfeeding: global sales in 2014 of US$44·8 billion show the industry's large, competitive claim on infant feeding' (Hansen, 2016).

When I was in Hong Kong, despite the protective benefits of breastfeeding being spoken of in the plenary session conference by a Nobel Prize winning scientist, delegates complained to the conference organisers that the morning tea was sponsored by a commercial baby milk manufacturer. The conference secretariats were more interested in the viability of the organisation and conference than the influence of advertising. Accepting the sponsorship reflected badly on the speaker, who had stated at the beginning of his presentation that he had no conflicts of interest. The speaker and breastfeeding advocates took their morning tea elsewhere but the damage was done.

My story: Papua New Guinea

In 1976, when working as a general nurse in PNG, I saw babies die from gastroenteritis due to being bottle-fed with breastmilk substitutes. Commercial baby milk was being promoted and sold at local supermarkets and trade stores to a population with minimal education and no understanding of bacteria. The villagers lived in grass huts without electricity or clean running water in a tropical environment that lacked adequate sanitation and refrigeration. Powdered milk is not a sterile product, and once opened in a humid climate, if not stored correctly can quickly grow bacteria and become lethal.

I was breastfeeding my four-month-old baby and bottle-feeding powdered milk to my toddler when we first arrived in PNG. A family member posted a cutting from *The Age* newspaper in Melbourne, listing the code numbers of the recalled brands of powdered milk I was using to feed my toddler. Pigeons had got into the factory in Australia and contaminated the product. On inspection by the local district health officer in PNG, a shipping container was found at the local port to contain some of the recalled milk, which was subsequently confiscated and destroyed.

Without fresh cow's milk in PNG, feeding a toddler was problematic. Our daughter suffered frequent episodes of diarrhoea. We sought medical help from a paediatrician from Rabaul, who had no solution. While visiting Port Moresby, we discovered when buying and consuming fresh imported cow's milk from a supermarket the diarrhoea stopped. It was the substituted powdered or tinned milk we were using because it was all that was available in Kimbe that had caused the diarrhoea. Had the paediatrician known or had we been enlightened about breastfeeding through our nursing or medical education, I would have expressed milk or tandem-fed our toddler.

Susanna I. Scurry

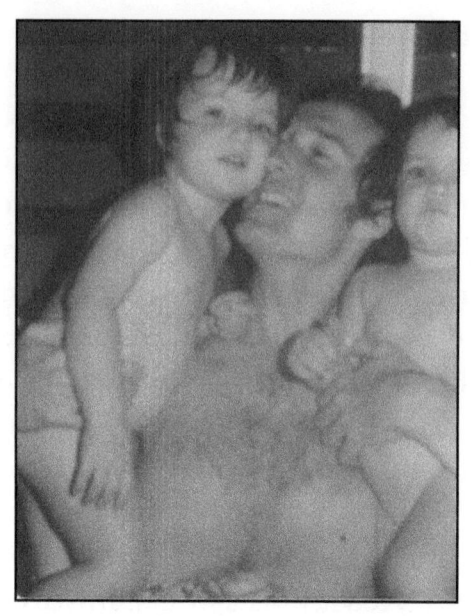

Jim and daughters, PNG, 1978

One of my strongest memories of PNG was an incident that occurred on our return from a hospital field trip. A storm blew up and we had to sit it out for around 24 hours as the outrigger was at risk of capsizing in the big waves. Upon arrival in Talasea, after remaining overnight on a sandbar, our bedraggled group was greeted by missionaries.

While we were waiting for the hospital transport, a missionary offered us bathing facilities to freshen up. As we walked to her home, a medical student from New Zealand who had accompanied us overheard the missionary chastising me for breastfeeding in front of the 'natives'. I was 24-years old and caring for a baby and toddler. I was exhausted and grateful I had been able to breastfeed the baby. I stood gobsmacked and totally humiliated. The medical student reacted quickly. Taking my arm and picking up the toddler, he turned us around and said to the woman that we no longer wanted a shower and would prefer to wait until we got home.

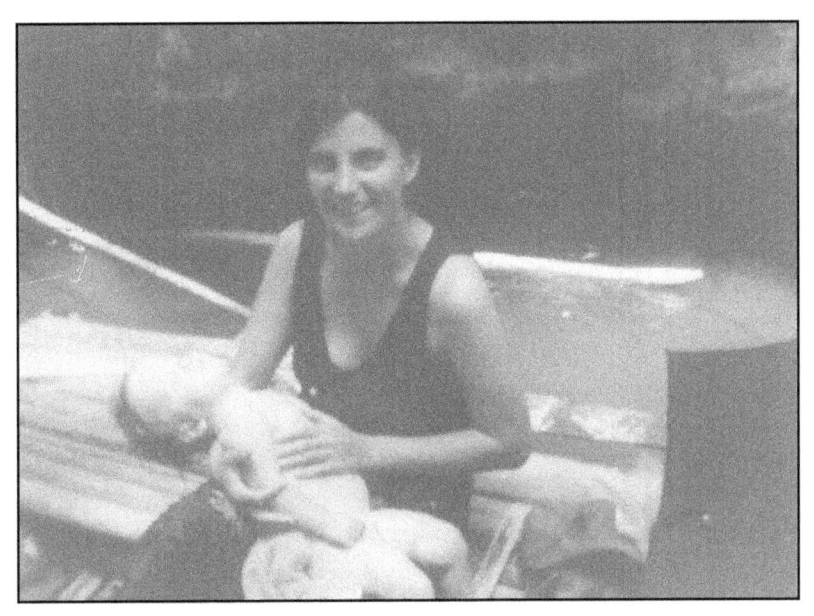

Jessica following a breastfeed and swim, PNG, 1977

PNG lags behind developed countries and a large majority of the rural population is uneducated and superstitious. The Health Department sent expatriates such as ourselves to rural areas and kept the locally trained graduates in the cities. During our stay in Kimbe, we went bushwalking with colleagues from the hospital, and they encouraged us to try eating the wild grapefruit. Twenty-four hours later, Jim, who had peeled the citrus, broke out in large blisters where the juice had spilt onto his hands. Where the juice had touched the children's skin when they had been picked up to be carried, they had large painful blisters the shape of handprints on their legs and trunk. The blisters were deep and resulted in permanent scarring. While recovering from the allergy at home, we were visited by a group of missionaries who had heard of our misfortune. They came with gifts of food. Like the priests of the past, they used superstition to create fear. They told me the allergy was caused by God and we were being punished for not heeding God's call. During our time in PNG, we also saw religious organisations using their position to exert power on villagers in outlying areas, denying children immunisations paid for by the government or schooling unless the parents attended church.

****

Abused and controlled

In the early 2000s, I attended a 'Women of Influence' luncheon in Sydney and heard Mary Robinson give a presentation. The former President of Ireland was the United Nations High Commissioner for Human Rights from 1997 to 2002. She stated human rights were at the heart of world peace, and structural changes were required to ensure that human rights were protected at every societal level. Mary Robinson is a staunch defender of gender equity. She believes the failure to hold those who abuse human rights accountable maintains a climate of impunity and exacerbates a sense of injustice and discrimination.

As a health professional, I am educated to recognise when women are being subjected to domestic abuse, of which there are many types. Coercive control includes patterns of behaviour or ways of manipulating relationships. The perpetrators of such control use strategic forms of behaviour and oppression to instil fear. Behaviours include isolating victims from support structures, using verbal or physical threats or violence, gas lighting, financial control, denying freedom and autonomy, and exploitative behaviours such as expecting women to go to work and then do an unequal share of the housework.

Historically, many of the features of coercive control have been used by patriarchal power groups to control women. In Australia, since colonisation, the country's leaders have reflected the cultural norms and religious views of the colonists which perpetuate outdated gender stereotyping and beliefs from the past and influence politicians and economists to reinforce gender stereotypes and expected behaviours.

Patriarchy, Misogyny and Breastfeeding

When poor Irish and English female prisoners arrived in Hobart in the nineteenth century, they were hired out by the prison authorities to clean the houses of the elite. Many were subjected to physical and sexual abuse by their employers. Women returning to prison pregnant were blamed, had their sentences prolonged by the length of the pregnancy and many babies died. The abusers were protected by the authorities.

Following the Second World War, women who had worked to support the war effort were required to give up their paid employment in favour of the returning men. Without a source of income, women were again dependant, and without a means of support many of them suffered. The Australian Human Rights Commission website lists ways women have been excluded from public and political life. Women were not elected to the Federal Parliament until 1943. Until the 1960s, women were forced to resign from their place of employment in the public service once they married. My aunt kept her marriage secret so she could continue to work as a teacher. And my mother, whose work was essential to the family business, was frequently the butt of prejudice from members of the community opposed to working women. Women were not permitted to drink in a public bar until 1965. I can remember the saloon bar being set aside for women when my parents bought a hotel, but I can also remember women sitting in the car outside patiently waiting for their men to finish drinking. The six o'clock swill, which ended shortly after my parents bought the hotel, was a disgusting exhibition of men finishing work and getting their fill of alcohol before the hotel closed at six o'clock.

My story: The horror of backyard abortionists

When I lived in East Melbourne during the 1980s and 90s, I had to pass a fertility clinic which had been set up by Doctor Bertram

Weiner in 1972. Prior to the clinic being opened, women died at the hands of backyard abortionists due to infection and bleeding after receiving a termination of pregnancy. They were too afraid to attend hospital emergency departments. Corrupt police, highly paid doctors, backyard abortionists and a conservative government supported by Catholic voters placed women in perilous situations, rather than providing them with safe and affordable family planning.

On an almost daily basis, I witnessed women entering and leaving the clinic being subjected to harassment by groups of religious right-to-life protestors. They gathered in front of the clinic holding up offensive placards, blocking the footpath and, on one occasion, murdering a security guard. During the same period of time, priests and church leaders were perpetrating sexual abuse against vulnerable children throughout the country and, in Australia at the time of writing, have not adequately been held to account.

****

In 2013, *The Guardian* reported that the police were complicit in enslaving 10,000 unmarried mothers across Ireland in laundries run by the Sisters of Charity. The McAleese Report found the women, called 'Maggies', worked unpaid in the Magdalene laundries, in some cases for life, because they were unmarried mothers and/or seen as morally wayward. In 2017, *The Guardian* also reported that following a public outcry, the Sisters of Charity who were complicit with the treatment of unmarried mothers announced that they were ending their role in the St Vincent's Health Care group and would not own or run the new National Maternity Hospital in Dublin.

In Australia, the treatment of unmarried mothers was not dissimilar. Some public maternity care is still run by the Catholic Church and can influence the care of women. For example, in my experience when women were seeking advice on the morning after pill they were directed to a non-Catholic institution. Another example of Catholic control involved caring for a mother who was bleeding due to a miscarriage. We were delayed in taking her to theatre until the blood test reported the pregnancy was no longer viable, despite the risk to the mother.

On 21 March 2013, Prime Minister Julia Gillard apologised on behalf of the Australian Government to 150,000 unmarried Australian mothers affected by forced adoption or removal policies and practices. Many books have been written by the women who had their babies taken from them. Lily McDonald's book, *Dirty Laundry*, speaks of her illegal imprisonment, cruel labour and the forced adoption of her son while under the care of nuns and state police in Queensland during the 1950s and 60s. Lily, as a pregnant teenager, was arrested, charged, sentenced and imprisoned in the Magdalene home for wayward girls in Wooloowin. She was forced to work without payment in the Magdalene's commercial laundry and her son was forcibly removed from her care, despite her partner having obtained signed formal permission to marry papers. He was denied contact with Lily and the Mother Superior refused to release her.

In Australia to this day, Catholic nuns and sisters have not been held accountable for the abuses against unmarried women and their babies. Mary Robinson pointed out in an address on human rights, 'A failure to ensure accountability can leave the most culpable of perpetrators in positions of power and able to exert malign influence. More generally, the lack of justice and accountability perpetuates a climate of impunity, which undermines the rule of law as well as exacerbating a sense of injustice and discrimination within targeted communities' (Robinson, 2002).

My story: religious control

In 1980, I began midwifery training at the Mercy Hospital for Women in East Melbourne. This was the same hospital I had left crying after being shamed by an obstetrician during my first antenatal visit appointment in 1975. While I was training, I witnessed the removal of infants from single women by the nuns. Great secrecy surrounded these cases, and the young mother was often discharged from hospital soon after the birth. The nuns were very much in control of these births and moved the babies to another area of the hospital away from their mother to be cared for by nurses in nurseries. The infants were rarely breastfed. Although mothers were given a period of time to change their minds, they were not encouraged to do so, and the power structures within the institution meant midwives did not interfere.

In 1975 and 76, I was an unmarried mother and subjected to the many prejudices of the time. As young parents we were unsure of ourselves but, at the same time, determined to keep our baby. We refused to be pushed around by anyone. After the experience at the first antenatal visit, we sought alternative maternity care and found a progressive female obstetrician whose only concern was that the baby was wanted. I delivered in a private hospital. However, my treatment at the hands of the midwives reflected the times and the hospital notes labelled me 'single girl keeping baby' (SGKB).

****

Misogyny at large

In Australia in 1982, Lindy Chamberlain was brought to trial after the disappearance of her baby daughter Azaria. All of Australia was abuzz with differing theories of what had occurred at Uluru

(Ayers Rock) and Lindy, Azaria's mother, was demonised by the press, hungry for news. I always believed the Chamberlain's account of the dingo taking baby Azaria. My uncle raised sheep and hated the dingoes, as during lambing season they would attack the lambs which, unlike baby Azaria, could run. At a school function one evening, I sat next to a lawyer who had worked on the prosecution case. When he spoke, I could feel his venom towards Lindy. I told the group how the dingoes behaved on my uncle's farm. The lawyer was furious with me, and to the group he said, 'I know she did it'. Rather than giving a reasoned response, he was a bully, shouting and clenching his fists while banging on the table. For whatever reason, this man hated women. And rather than treat Lindy as a poor mother who had lost her baby, he wanted to punish her. Lindy was eventually released from prison three years later and subsequently pardoned when a crucial piece of evidence (Azaria's matinee jacket) was found at Uluru.

As long as there is gender imbalance in the law, policing and corrective services, resources may be directed away from protection and care of women. It was lack of resources that allowed the violent rampage of the 'Parramatta bomber' to go on for 15 years before he was apprehended. He was responsible for several murders and eventually convicted of murdering a family court judge, bombing a Jehovah's Witness church where parishioners died, and bombing the family court in Parramatta (while being suspected of crimes not proven) and sentenced to a long jail term. The Parramatta bomber was a controlling husband who perpetrated crimes against anyone who provided support to his former partner, including her brother, whose body has never been found.

In Melbourne, Victoria, on 10 March 2023, *The Guardian* reported that a male judge had asked a breastfeeding mother to leave the court because breastfeeding was distracting for court occupants. That afternoon, when visiting a friend, I asked her husband, an elderly, and boys' school-educated lawyer, what he thought of the judge's behaviour. He went on a tirade, saying he fully supported the judge's direction, making lewd comments about jurors ogling the women's breasts and being distracted. He said it was obscene to have a child suckling on a woman's breasts, rather than listening to points of law, and had he been on the case and lost, he would have appealed to the Supreme Court. Breastfeeding within Australia's legal system remains in the Dark Ages, with women prisoners' babies being denied the right to be breastfed. The legal system continues to see optimum nutrition as non-essential.

Australian prisons do have mother and baby units designed to keep mothers and infants together. However, in a lecture at an Australian Breastfeeding Association study day, academic and researcher Karleen Gribble stated that women requesting to remain with their babies while incarcerated is a cumbersome process, and accessing facilities is difficult.

Oxytocin is known as the 'hormone of love' and released during breastfeeding. Because oxytocin facilitates bonding and caring behaviours of parents, keeping mothers with their infants should be a priority. Government, law enforcement and the legal profession have failed Australian women and children since Australia was colonised. The English adversarial system brought with the colonists requires victims to relive their abuse and perpetuates the trauma they have experienced.

When travelling to different parts of the industrialised world, I am made aware of how vast distance is a disadvantage to the dissemination of ideas, and how the lack of diversity in the Australian media hinders intelligent debate. In Australia, the human body and sex continues to be a cause for embarrassment and treated as suspect, both inside and outside of marriage. Young people are subjected to sad and outdated views and, rather than being given accurate information, have restrictions placed on what is normal sexual behaviour. Ideologies from the past perpetuate untruths, rather than keep the young safe. I was astounded when my cousin's children were discussing male circumcision, which they believed would protect them from venereal disease. When I challenged them and suggested they use a condom for protection from both venereal disease and an unwanted pregnancy, they were surprised. Our young need to be educated in schools and universities that teach evidence-based science so they are not left defenceless because of outdated ideologies.

In my work at the hospital, mandatory education policies teach staff to behave towards others as you would treat a family member or wish to be treated yourself. While there are times when dealing with sick or mentally unwell clients may be difficult, adhering to the human rights principles as listed on the Australian Human Rights Commission is helpful. A young, new lactation consultant I know was concerned about changes to infant feeling guidelines and what to tell the parents. She thought the ambiguity within the guidelines may push the mother in a way she considered inappropriate. My response was that her job was to give the current and evidence-based information and respect the mother's decision no matter what she decided.

Human rights recognise the inherent value of each person, regardless of background, where they live, what they look like, what they think or what they believe. Human rights are based on principles of dignity, equity and mutual respect, which is shared across cultures, religions and philosophies. Human rights are about being treated fairly, treating others fairly and having the ability to make genuine choices in our daily lives. Respect for human rights is the cornerstone of strong communities in which everyone can make a contribution and feel included.

3

A History of Birthing

The history of medicine and birthing has been well documented, as has the history of infant feeding. The oldest university in the world is the University of Al Quaraouiyine, which was established in Fez, Morocco in the year 859. The first medical school began in Italy at the University of Bologna in 1219, followed in Britain by the University of Oxford. Women were excluded from a university education, and the gender-specific nature of birth and breastfeeding left maternity to midwives and women. University-educated physicians received an education that evolved from the fifth century and was based on theory, supposition and superstition.

Physicians were not permitted to practise without permission from a priest, and medical training could never be in conflict with Church doctrine. Unfortunately, the Catholic Church was interested in saving souls and the afterlife, rather than in the relief of suffering or healing the body. Men who entered physician training were often priests whose beliefs forbade them to deal with blood.

Training for physicians was limited to purging and leeches. Writings and cartoons of the time often portray physicians as pumped up, overdressed charlatans, with little to offer that may have been of comfort. Microorganisms such as bacteria and viruses were not discovered until the nineteenth century, and physicians believed that a miasma (ill wind) or the wrath of the gods caused illnesses.

There was no understanding of the impact of lack of hygiene, nor the ramifications of pollution and poverty on health.

A feminist perspective

In 1973, Barbara Ehenreich and Deirdre English wrote a feminist perspective entititled *Witches, Midwives and Nurses*, and presented reasons for the lack of women healers. The authors argued that the upper classes were in a position to pay the fees demanded by physicians and were afraid of midwives and women healers, who charged low fees and had power, knowledge and the experience to relieve suffering. As time evolved, the medical profession was in direct competition with these independent women, and were compicit in the 'witch hunts' that lasted from the fourteenth to the seventeenth century. Although proof is difficult to obtain, historian John Demos estimates that between 50,000 and 100,000 so-called witches were executed during the witch hunts by the Catholic Church, and 85 per cent of them were women healers and midwives (Demos, 2008).

When I visited Edinburgh, I took a tour of the city. As the tour group walked up the hill to Edinburgh Castle, the guide asked all those wearing orange to stand to one side. He told the tour group that during the sixteenth, seventeenth and eighteenth centuries, a woman wearing orange could be accused of being a witch and would be placed in a barrel and rolled down Castlehill Edinburgh Road. Any woman who survived the ordeal was then burned at the stake as a witch, while those who died were declared innocent. The women healers' crimes were female sexuality, magical powers and being organised.

In many cultures, men were repulsed by 'birth dirt' and women's leaking bodies, and required women to be separated from the group during times of bleeding. Historically, religious leaders harnessed the fear of contagion to control populations, and purification rituals such as baptism remain common religious ceremonies today.

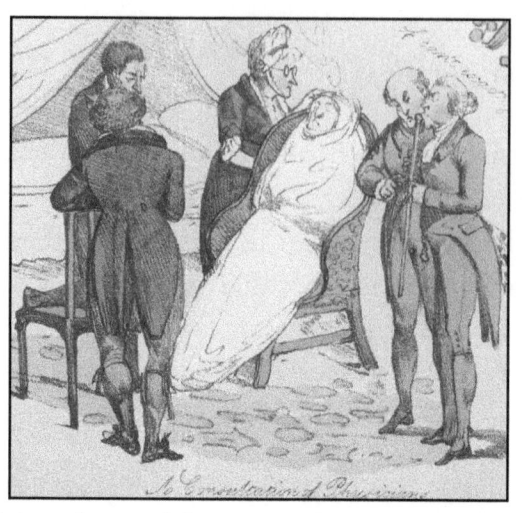

A Consultation of Physicians, unknown artist, ©Royal College of Physicians, photography by John Chase

Men and medicine

The elite and wealthier upper classes who were afraid of the poor and could afford the cost were attended by university-educated physicians. Surgeons, unlike their physician counterparts who avoided physical contact with clients and blood, were more practical. They gained their knowledge through experience, either working in hospitals or travelling with armies and learning on the battlefields. How infection was spread was not understood, and neither handwashing nor cleanliness was considered. Barber surgeons in Britain performed minor operations such as tooth extractions and bone setting, with their main occupation cutting or shaving hair.

Apothecaries were on the lowest rung of the medical hierarchy, with the highest number of practitioners. Originally, they were grocers concocting – often dubious – potions. Over time, they became more specialised and were the original general practitioners, giving medical advice and drugs, and providing low-cost services to the bulk of the population.

When physicians, surgeons and apothecaries sought a larger share of the market, they were able to have laws put in place to govern their profession and exclude women. The differences between the three groups are important because the lower status groups gained power from their amalgamation with the physicians and their upper-class contacts. The *UK Medical Act* 1858 (duplicated in Australia soon after) brought together physicians, surgeons and apothecaries, and gave medicine the right to control other health practitioners. Independent midwives were excluded because obstetrical forceps were legally classified as surgical instruments, which could only be used by surgeons. The medicalisation of birth in Australia followed a similar trajectory to that in Britain (Fahy, 2007).

Midwife care

Author and French obstetrician Michel Odent hypothesised that the probable historical origin of midwifery is rooted in preliterate and preagricultural societies, with members of the birthing women's family protecting the birthing space from wild animals or men (Odent, 2009). Women, like most mammals, birthed in isolation in the bush or in a special birthing hut.

Over the millennia, birth became socialised and birthing women were cared for by other women or midwives at home. Women's leaking bodies were seen as a form of pollution that could cause contagion, and were managed by other women. Women, being denied formal education, learned through experience or gained skills passed from one generation to the next.

In Britain, in the early to mid-nineteenth century, some general practitioners immigrated to Australia due to competition at home.

They settled mainly in the cities, where they set up medical practices. Without scientific evidence, general practitioners had little claim to expert knowledge and had difficulty in gaining a competitive advantage over independent midwives, who were held in high regard until the 1880s and considered valued members of the community.

During the pioneering era from 1820 to 1880, due to a lack of doctors in rural areas, many independent midwives set up private lying-in homes or hospitals. Near Bellingen, NSW, a converted home was once a maternity hospital run by an independent midwife. Built on a hillside with sweeping views and large rooms opening onto wide verandas, it offered a restful space for women to recuperate following the births of their babies while receiving help from a midwife. At my home in Stockton, before the bridge was built over the Hunter River in 1971, many elderly residents were birthed by the local resident midwife in a beautiful old home on the main street, with balcony rooms looking out over the Pacific Ocean.

Childbirth and male practitioners

'Man-midwife' was a term used to describe specialist males birthing women prior to the 1930s, and they were different from traditional independent female midwives. The main reasons for the rise in popularity of the man-midwife were knowledge, fashion and forceps, which was their point of difference from the traditional midwife. While normal birth was the domain of female midwives, occasionally a surgeon was required to use surgical instruments if labour was obstructed. Only qualified surgeons were legally permitted to use forceps and only a man could be educated to become a surgeon, or perform a Caesarean section if the mother had died and there was a chance of saving the baby. At the end of the eighteenth century, surgeon-apothecaries, who were all but general practitioners in name, attended home births when a midwife was unavailable or the patient requested the doctor be there.

Lying-in hospitals were first established in the eighteenth century and between 1730 and 1930 were a serious risk for parturient women due to infection, with major outbreaks of puerperal sepsis closely linked to the practice of man-midwives. Lying-in hospitals had three aims.

- To deliver poor women free of charge.
- To provide access and experience for medical, male accoucheurs/man-midwives to deliver a large number of babies.
- To provide a convenient central point for man-midwives, who could attend more patients and undermine the customer base of independent midwives.

In 1740, William Smellie, a Scottish man-midwife, set up a lying-in hospital in London for the poor. Smellie used forceps he had designed made of metal and covered in leather, making them difficult to clean. In an article published in 2012 in the *Journal of Obstetrics and Gynaecology*, Doctor DC Shelton questioned the continuing 'approbation of William Smellie and William Hunter [a student of Smellie] as "Founding Fathers" of the obstetrics profession' (Shelton, 2012).

> ... the worth of man-midwifery do not stand up to forensic scrutiny. Combining the legacy of extra maternal and neonatal deaths, together with subjects murdered for dissection, derives around 1 million human deaths connected to man-midwifery initiatives of the 18th century. In simple terms, those deaths arose from dismantling the pre-1730 structure of maternal home-care provided by trained midwives ... Such

censure would then avoid their unethical practices tainting the positive achievements of the obstetrics profession in the 80 years since 1929.

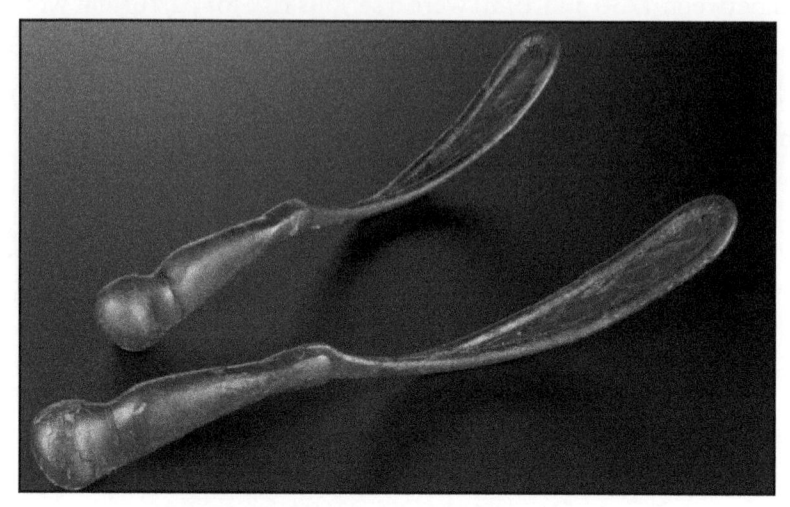

Eighteenth-century obstetric metal and leather forceps designed by William Smellie, Science Museum, London

In 1852, the maternal death rate for women who died at home in childbirth in Glasgow was one woman in 325 births, compared to the death rate of one woman in 77 births in lying-in hospitals run by man-midwives (see Figure 3.1).

Figure 3.1: Comparison of maternal deaths in Glasgow, Scotland 1720–1930: Blue physician/hospital MMR/10,000; red mwife/GP home births MMR ratio. Source: DC Shelton, 2012

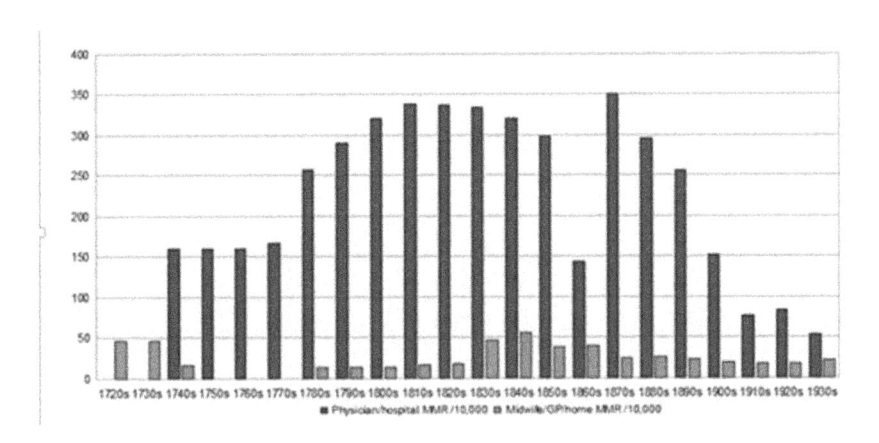

In 1856, The Royal Women's Hospital was established in East Melbourne, as the Lying-in Hospital and Infirmary for Diseases Peculiar to Women and Children. The hospital was set up by a committee of women led by Mrs Frances Perry, the wife of the Anglican bishop of Melbourne. She was supported by Doctor Richard Tracy, who graduated from the Dublin School of Medicine in 1848, and Doctor John Maund who had gained his qualifications from the University of Glasgow and the Royal College of Surgeons. Doctor Tracy had immigrated to Australia in 1851. He practised in Adelaide before going to Castlemaine and Bendigo where gold had been discovered to seek his fortune. However, he became tired of life on the goldfields and moved onto Melbourne where he began practising medicine again.

The impact of Florence Nightingale in Australia

When still a British colony, Australia's first nurses came in response to a request from Governor Parkes to Florence Nightingale. In March

1868, six nurses sent by Nightingale arrived in Sydney. Since the arrival of the colonists, Australian hospitals had been run by military doctors and were poorly managed, plagued by scandal, dirty and overrun by rats. One of the nurses, Lucy Osburn, was appointed superintendent of the Sydney Infirmary and Dispensary. She worked hard to reform the hospitals but faced stiff opposition from the colony's doctors. She is reputed to have set up Sydney's first nursing school in Macquarie Street.

Nursing had emerged as an occupational group from the Crimean War (1854–1856). Nightingale, when working in military hospitals during the war, saw more soldiers in hospitals die as a result of their injuries than on the battlefield. Florence Nightingale belonged to the English upper class and used her influence, and statistical evidence, to bring about change. Her essays, *Notes on Hospitals* (1859), emphasised the importance of cleanliness and hygiene prior to the acceptance of 'germ theory' in the 1890s.

The hospital model set up by Nightingale was based on a military model, with nurses subordinate to doctors. She believed birthing women should be kept separate from hospitalised patients. As a statistician, she recognised the dangers of lying-in hospitals, where many women died from puerperal fever due to overcrowding, unwashed instruments, contaminated linen and a high frequency of internal examinations.

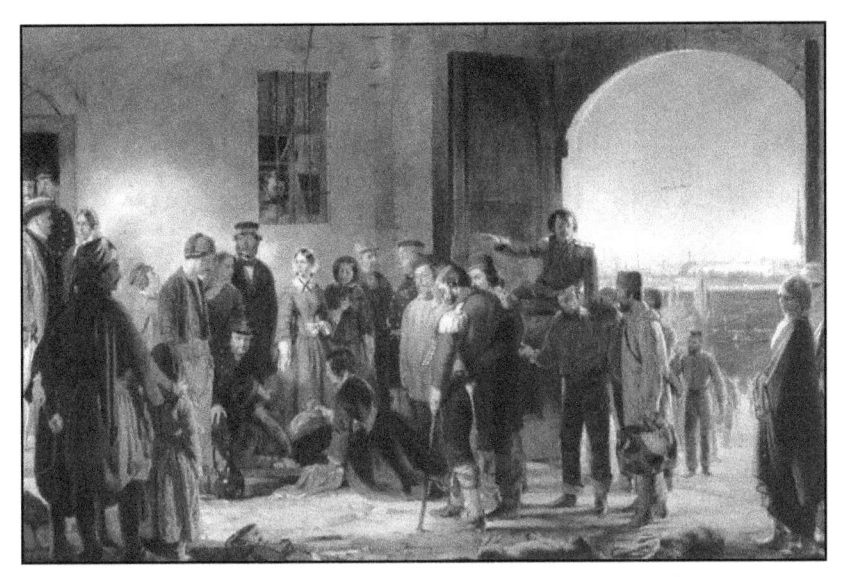

Florence Nightingale receiving the wounded at Scuteri during the Crimean War, Jerry Barrett, 1856, National Portrait Gallery, London

Doctors and nurses in alliance

When doctors and nurses in both the United Kingdom and Australia forged an alliance between 1886 and 1928, the coming together of the two groups placed hospital care of women outside the realms of independent midwives. Both medicine and nursing used their power to ensure that the Diploma of Midwifery could only be taken by women who had completed their general nursing training. The Royal Women's Hospital in Melbourne commenced midwifery training in 1888, placing midwives under the control of predominately university-educated male physicians.

In 1896, the Queen Victoria Hospital was set up by 11 female doctors led by Doctor Constance Stone, who had travelled to the United States in 1884 to obtain her medical qualification. Women were not admitted to The University of Melbourne to study medicine until 1887. After graduating, female doctors found it difficult to obtain employment in the Melbourne hospital system as they were not welcomed by the male Victorian medical establishment. The hospital was set up to treat poor women uncomfortable in the care of male doctors, and the hospital was run by women, for women and children. The monies raised to build the Queen Vic came from a public appeal called the 'Shilling Fund'. As well as care, the hospital provided training and employment for the small but increasing number of women doctors.

Hospital care in Australia

Australian hospital design was based on the English model. Women in lower socio-economic groups who could not afford to pay for a private doctor or a single room were housed in shared wards. Maternity hospital postnatal wards copied the acute hospital design with nurseries being built and babies separated from their mothers where they were cared for by nurses and midwives.

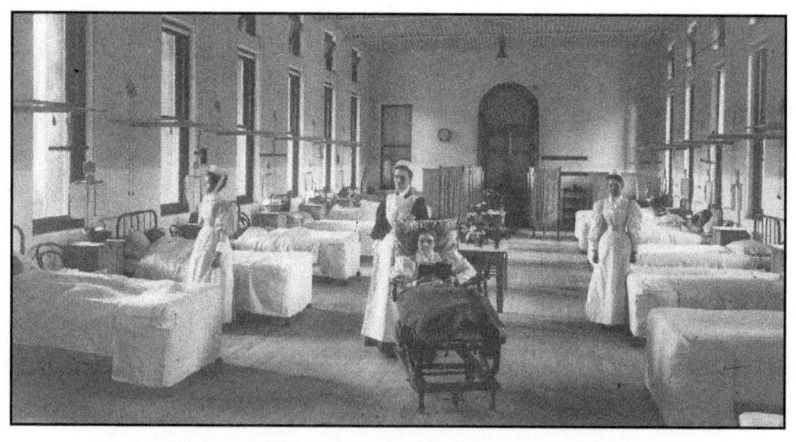

Interior of the women's surgical ward, Sydney Hospital, 1890s. National Museum Australia. Note the similarities between this ward and maternity ward in the illustration on the next page.

Traditionally, most public hospitals placed women in open wards, with portable curtains offering minimal privacy. Babies were separated from their mothers and cared for by nurses and midwives in nurseries. Many current public postnatal wards remain little changed from their original design, with women in two- or four-bed rooms, with shared bathrooms and toilets. In BFHI-accredited hospitals, where infants room in with their mothers, nurseries for well babies on the postnatal wards have been closed.

Shared rooms are not appropriate for postnatal women, especially given the gender-specific nature of birth and breastfeeding. A family member cannot remain after visiting hours to help, and being separated by curtains makes it difficult to maintain adequate privacy and confidentiality, or create a quiet space to allow the mother to rest. However, they continue to be used, not only because they are cost-effective but also because the private medical model has a vested interest in weakening the competition between the public and private hospital systems.

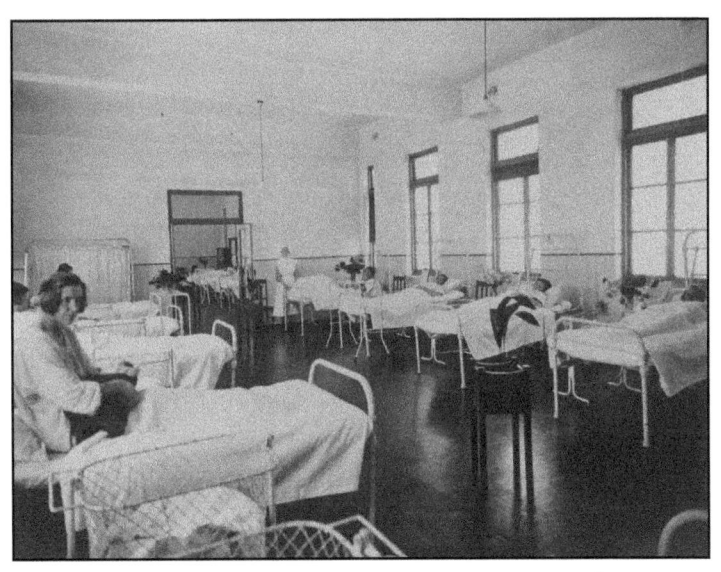

Crown Street Women's Hospital maternity ward c.1920s. City of Sydney Archives, 2023

In Australian hospitals, the English class system was perpetuated with hierarchical structures put in place. The doctors were in charge, nursing care was provided by women who were subordinate to the doctors and had little autonomy, and snobbery was rife. Women from lower socio-economic groups were cared for by the junior doctors and medical students, and supervised by the senior doctors with university appointments. The senior consultants were like gods, as they had the power to hire or fire and pass or fail those studying within the system.

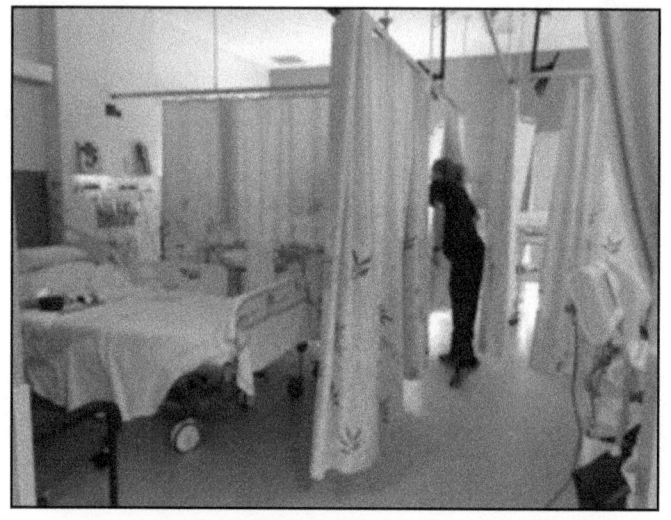

A four-bed postnatal ward where mothers and infants are separated by curtains in a NSW public hospital, 2021

Once women in hospitals were placed under the control of doctors and birth medicalised, the ultimate need of the woman as mother was lost. Postnatal care and the optimum wellbeing and recovery of the mother has been on the lowest rung of the hospital childbirth hierarchy for decades. Once the baby is born, care of the mother passes to midwives who are at the lower end of the hierarchy and trained to support the doctors. The focus of postnatal care is post-operative care and the recognition of medical complications such as infection.

In the current hospital model women barely have time to rest and recover from birth before being discharged, often to manage with minimum support. The different psychological phases of mothering are not considered. Having time to develop skills and confidence in both mothering and breastfeeding are of little interest to most doctors.

Post-war changes

Following the Second World War in Australia, the resultant baby boom filled hospitals and new maternity services were required. Many technologies had been improved during the war, and the development of antibiotics, improvements in pain relief and anaesthetics, and the use of blood transfusions had a great impact. Women who would have previously died from infection or blood loss were able to be saved and the dangers posed by operative births and infection decreased.

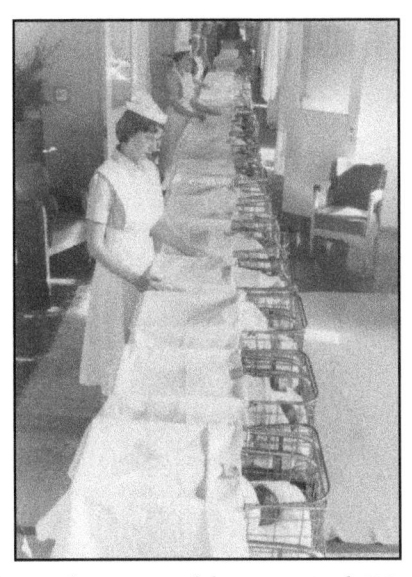

Nurses caring for babies in the nursery of the Henry Pride Wing, added to The Royal Women's Hospital in 1958 as a result of the baby boom, which followed the end of the Second World War. Source: The Royal Women's Hospital archival collection

In the past, the point of difference between midwives and man-midwives, who had a name change in Australia to obstetrician in the 1930s, was knowledge and legalisation of surgical equipment. Currently, without the complications of the past and increased incentives to perform a caesarean section, normal vaginal birth rates have decreased. More women are having surgical interventions and left caring for a baby after shorter hospital stays and with less help. However, despite the advances in science, caesarean section is not without risk, and women are left with scarring on the uterus after the procedure. This creates another dimension to obstetric care because of the added risk of conditions such as placenta accreta in a subsequent pregnancy. This is a serious complication of pregnancy and can cause severe blood loss, sometimes requiring a hysterectomy. Care of women with a placenta accreta requires highly skilled professionals. I was at a research meeting where the research obstetrician was keen to try to preserve a patient's uterus by leaving the imbedded placenta attached to it. As the birth was likely to be the woman's last, I raised the fact that the woman would be unlikely to breastfeed, as it is the empty uterus that initiates an adequate amount of breastmilk. The obstetrician had failed to consider the importance of breastfeeding to the mother.

My Aunty Bonnie trained as a midwife in Brisbane during the 1950s. After her death, I was given her hospital nursery routine notes, which described the regimented care provided by midwives.

- The nursery temperature was to be maintained at 100 degrees Fahrenheit.
- All new babies are to be supervised at first breastfeeding.
- Report any difficult babies to Sister in Charge.
- Mothers' nipples to be washed with Boracic Acid solution 1–40, before and after feeds, and dried.
- 1st day: 4-hourly 3 by 3 minutes at breast.
- 2nd day: 4-hourly 7 by 7 minutes at breast.

- 3rd day: 4-hourly 10 by 10 minutes at breast.
- Test feed and complement. Babies must be weighed on the back in centre of scales.
- 4th day and thereafter: the Sister in Charge will determine time and amount according to mother's lactation.
- Mothers to have a breast binder on the third day. If their breasts are engorged, foments (warm bathe) before feed and hot water bags between feeds.

My story: midwifery training

I trained to be a midwife after the birth of my third child. My training was inspired by the work of the Melanesian midwives I had seen while living in PNG.

In the spring of 1980, I joined a tightknit group of students, including one male, and commenced the 12-month midwifery training program at the Mercy Hospital for Women in East Melbourne. As registered nurses, we already had skills and were immediately rostered to work on the wards. As a young mother, I empathised with the women.

I worked shift work, which included morning, evening and night duty. We worked in most areas of the hospital, including the delivery suite, antenatal outpatient, the postnatal wards, the neonatal nursery and the milk room. Blocks of lectures and exams were scheduled throughout the year. Much emphasis was placed on screening the women and detection of potential issues that could impact the birth, labour and delivery. We were taught the mechanisms of normal birth and how to deliver an infant without damage to the perineum but birth was not sacred and how breastfeeding could prevent haemorrhage or help contract the uterus were all minimised by what Michel Odent calls the masculinisation of birth (Odent, 2009).The focus of the course was on recognition of deviations from normal birthing and when to intervene.

Hospitals that are BFHI accredited had not been introduced, and babies were cared for in the nursery. Babies could remain with their mothers during the day but returned to the nursery overnight and at rest times, where they were cared for by mothercraft nurses trained under the scientific mothering principles of Doctor (later Sir) Truby King (see also Chapter 7).

I worked full-time throughout the 12 months and was paid a wage, which I used to remunerate a childcare worker that we had hired to care for the three children at home. As my husband was working full-time, it was easier for us all. The morning shift began at 7:00 am, finishing at 3.30 pm; the afternoon shift at 1:30 pm finishing at 10:00 pm. Night shift began at 9.30 pm and finished the following morning at 7:30 am. Weekend work was also required. The children liked being at home. My husband was home in the evenings and he preferred to be with the children without the babysitter, who would leave early or not come in, without any change to her wage. After my tax and paying the carer there was nothing left. One afternoon two hours before I was to start an afternoon shift, the babysitter telephoned to say she was ill. I was unable to replace her at such short notice and telephoned work to explain that I could not leave the children. Upon returning to work the following day, I was reprimanded by the nun in charge and told, if the incident was repeated, I would be sacked. The nuns showed little sympathy for mothers. It would have been better had I lied and said I was sick as I completed midwifery having used none of the allocated five days of sick leave.

Although I loved my midwifery training – the mothers and babies, the course work and the friends I made – I found the hierarchical, patriarchal, religious and inequitable care of the women confronting. Privately insured women had continuity of care with their chosen obstetricians and a single or double room, which allowed for rest and privacy. They were fawned over by the obstetricians and nuns. Meanwhile, the public women were kept waiting in the often-cold antenatal outpatient ward in degrading white gowns for long periods to see different junior doctors or consultant obstetricians and students each visit. Obstetricians with private patients often left junior doctors to complete the work and they did not complain as their future jobs or exam results may have been jeopardised. Midwives did as they were instructed.

In the labour ward, medical students and student midwives competed to care for the birthing women, with obstetricians favouring the medical students. All students were required to witness ten births before being permitted to undertake a baby's delivery, and all students needed to undertake ten deliveries to obtain their qualification. When a delivery was imminent, the bells would ring, and an announcement could be heard over the hospital intercom. Those students fastest and with the sharpest elbows were ushered into the labouring woman's room as she was about to birth. Students would observe from the back of the room. If the woman was a private patient and the obstetrician and woman agreed, one or two students were invited to witness the birth, while the public woman may have had up to five or more students in the room at one time. Having already given birth to three children, I realised that the invasion of the birthing space by strangers was degrading for many women. Women often said, 'Leave your modesty at the front door and pick it up on the way out'.

Students were also required to witness two caesarean births as part of their training. During one of the births I attended, I was horrified to see the consultant obstetrician using the anaesthetised woman to demonstrate a vaginal examination before the operation commenced. Around ten medical students, one after the other, practised performing a vaginal examination on the woman under the consultant obstetrician's instruction. To this day, I feel shame that

I did not complain. However, like many other trainees, I was fearful of the consequences for my career.

For one week we worked in the milk room, making up milk for differing babies' requirements in the hospital. Leftover expressed breastmilk from the mothers was pooled and used for other mothers' babies in the nursery. We understood how precious breastmilk was for the infants within the NICU and never wasted a drop. The use of other mothers' milk was used in neonatal nurseries until everything stopped due to risk of transmission of infection when the AIDS pandemic occurred.

The East Melbourne Mercy was an innovative design. Visitors entered the mother's room from an outside corridor, which was between the hospital windows and the rooms. The large windows provided light and sweeping views over the Fitzroy Gardens and Melbourne. The nurses and doctors entered the nurses' stations from a central corridor.

I had my fourth child soon after completing my midwifery training, as I was ready and wanted another baby. The baby boy was born at ten in the evening. We were thrilled, as we now had two boys and two girls, and the birth had been quick and easy. Jim and I wanted to remain together with the baby to celebrate. However, I was transferred to a shared waiting-room outside the delivery suite for several hours, and Jim could not stay due to the inappropriate environment where women were within close proximity and separated only by curtains. Keeping parents together to bond with the baby as a family was not a high priority in the 1980s. Although I had private insurance and a single room because I wanted my children to visit and not cause a disturbance to other women, I was disappointed in the way my baby's father was excluded during the crucial bonding period.

I decided that the delivery of our last three children would be under the care of an obstetrician in hospital. I chose him because he had a reputation for supporting normal birth and was respected because of his wisdom and experience. The option to have continuity of care with an independent midwife was problematic because at that time it was difficult to obtain support inside the hospital system when birth deviated from normal and a woman needed extra hospitalised care, for example when a haemorrhage occurred. Even today, when women choose a home birth and problems arise, hospitals and doctors are not always helpful. It is all about control. When I was training to be a midwife there was a private obstetrician who birthed women at home in the outer suburbs of Melbourne and he was constantly bad-mouthed and harassed by his colleagues.

When I finally arrived in the postnatal ward, a midwifery friend from my training school was on night duty. My baby had fed well following birth in the delivery suite, and I expected him to have a hibernation sleep, which is normal for a healthy-term infant. I did not want any top-ups of milk to be given in the nursery, and I trusted my friend when she told me she would bring the baby to me when he woke if I let her care for him in the nursery. She returned him to me at 5 am and I breastfed him to WHO recommendations.

4

The Changing Nature of Birthing

In November 2023, the *Australia's Mothers and Babies Report* in Australia reported that 315,705 babies were born to 311,360 mothers in 2021. A total of 62 per cent of mothers (192,392) had a vaginal birth and 38 per cent (118,887) had a caesarean section. Less than half of all births were non-instrumental vaginal births. When instrumental births were required, ventouse or vacuum extraction was more common (7.2 per cent) than forceps (4.8 per cent).

According to the report there are around 1000 different models of maternity care in use in 251 hospitals around the country. The public hospital care model accounted for 41 per cent of births, with most babies born in hospitals in conventional labour wards (96 per cent). A total of 29 per cent of women birth within a continuity of care arrangement, while 36 per cent have no continuity of carer.

A total of 75 per cent of women birthed within the publicly funded hospital system. The average number of days, women spent in hospital following childbirth steadily declined to two and a half days in 2021 from three days in 2011. Mothers were most likely to be discharged home between two and four days after giving birth: 65 per cent in 2010 and 62 per cent in 2021 (Australian Institute of Health and Welfare, 2023a). First-time mothers, those aged 40 years or more, women who had a preterm birth, multiple babies and women who had a caesarean section are likely to have longer stays of four days or more.

The report records that, in 2021, 108,909 (38 per cent) of women had a caesarean section compared to 32 per cent in 2011. Of those, 51,792 women had a previous caesarean section, the commonest reason for a repeat operation, 24 per cent had one previous caesarean section, 5.7 per cent had experienced two previous caesarean sections, and 1.5 per cent had three or more operative births. The report stated the caesarean section rate was 43 per cent in private hospitals compared to 29 per cent in the public sector.

First-time mothers made up 33 per cent of women who had a caesarean section. Caesarean section was more common among women whose babies were preterm, mothers older than 40 years, and mothers who were overweight.

In 2017, Australia's caesarean section rate was higher than the OECD average, ranking 27th out of 34 OECD countries, with a rate of 33.7 per 100 live births. Figure 4.1 demonstrates the declining rate of normal vaginal birth rate in Australia.

Figure 4.1: Type of delivery at birth in Australia, 2021. Source: Australian Institute of Health and Welfare

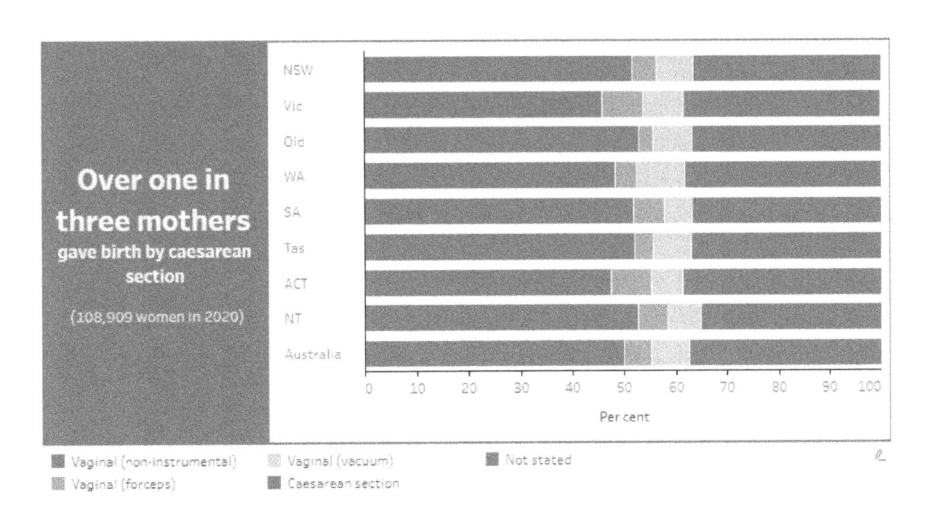

The Royal Australian and New Zealand College of Obstetricians and Gynaecologists describes a caesarean section as an operation where a baby is born through an incision made through the mother's abdomen and uterus. A caesarean section is generally performed when vaginal delivery is likely to pose a risk to the health of the mother or baby. The report recognises that a caesarean section can be associated with an increased danger for women and their babies during subsequent pregnancies.

My story: Risk with caesarean section

I had a colleague working during the night in the emergency department of a large maternity hospital, where a mother was admitted in labour. The woman had previously undergone a caesarean section. The labour ward was busy, no beds were available, and the medical team was in the operating theatre with another woman. The midwife was instructed to administer pain relief and observe the woman. She notified the labour ward staff that the labour was progressing and the woman's pain was worse. When the woman was finally seen, the uterus had ruptured and the baby had died.

I was present at an audit meeting when the deaths of three babies were being evaluated. The elephant in the room was the scarring on each woman's uterus from previous caesarean births. If there are no doctors available to perform a timely repeat caesarean section, there is little a midwife can do to prevent the contractions causing the scarring on the uterus to rupture. While in the Kimbe hospital I only saw two caesarean sections performed by the doctors due to the risks posed by scarring on the uterus in subsequent pregnancies. All women at risks, including those with uterine scarring, were transferred to Rabaul prior to the birth. Most mothers had a normal vaginal birth or ventouse (assisted delivery) delivery in PNG.

****

Impact of caesarean section on breastfeeding

Prevention of unnecessary caesarean section through the support of normal birth programs is important. One Australian research study asked thousands of women, 'Would you do anything different if you were to have another baby?' and reported over 85 per cent of women left comments related to making different decisions regarding their next birth choices (Keedle, 2023 et al). The study found women often blamed themselves for not being more informed and realised the benefits of continuity of care with a midwife. Many women also desired a vaginal birth as well as better access to birthing at home. Women who choose to give birth vaginally after having had a previous caesarean section are successful under the right circumstances.

Caesarean section birth rates continue to rise worldwide. A 2016 study reported caesarean section rates of 24.5 per cent in Western Europe, 32 per cent in North America and 41 per cent in South America (Betrán, 2016 et al). Caesarean section is a recognised cause for reduced breastfeeding outcomes (COAG, 2019).

Babies of mothers born following caesarean section may experience breastfeeding difficulties due to the lack of expulsion of amniotic fluid and mucus from the gut (see Figure 4.2). These babies are prone to gagging and vomiting and may not want to feed until they have expelled their gut contents, which normally occurs within the first 24 to 48 hours. Both mothers and midwives may become anxious and introduce commercial baby milk during this period.

Another impact of a caesarean section on breastfeeding mothers can be a delay in the onset of lactogenesis two, that is the copious production of breastmilk, which usually occurs around three days after birth. This can be caused by stress, a long labour prior to the caesarean section, a more than normal blood loss, or underlying conditions such as diabetes. Without correct knowledge and implementing practices to stimulate the mother's own milk, a mother may come to depend upon the commercial baby milk because of her pain and fatigue and lose her own supply.

Figure 4.2: Exclusive and partial breastfeeding rates compared with commercial milk feeding from 2007–2019 in women following caesarean section at hospital discharge. Source: NSW Ministry of Health

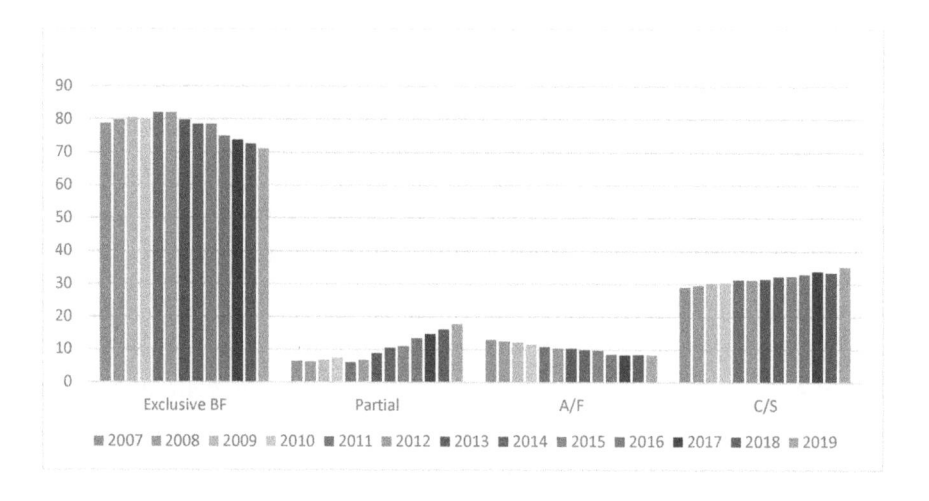

One of the key messages from a study in the United Kingdom was, 'Policy makers in settings with high rates of caesarean birth need to consider shorter and longer-term consequences for maternal and infant health if breastfeeding support is not addressed as a priority, particularly for women giving birth who have physical and/or psychological co-morbidity' (Beake et al, 2017).

Babies born following intrapartum administration of intravenous fluids during a caesarean section may take on extra fluids due to the volume of fluids administered to the mother during the operation or anaesthetic. Healthcare providers use infant's weight loss in the first days of life as a measurement of effective breastfeeding. Without adequate time or skills to assess these mothers and infants, mothers, midwives or nurses may become concerned by the more than normal weight loss and refer the infant to the neonatal unit or introduce artificial baby milk. The babies, like their mothers, having received extra IV fluid, will urinate extra fluid within the first few days following birth and appear to have excessive weight loss. These babies, instead of typically having one wet nappy in the first 24 hours following birth, may have two or three. Time, as well as adequately skilled staff, is required to ensure that the reasons for the weight loss is fully understood.

Hospital protocols may require infants losing more than 7 per cent of their birth weight to be referred to the neonatal team. This may result in doctors prescribing commercial baby milk top-ups, which undermines breastfeeding. Giving the top-ups can also result in the baby vomiting or requiring longer periods to sleep between feeds to digest the milk. While providing blessed relief for parents, this can reduce breastfeeding hormone levels and the mother's breastmilk supply. An American breastfeeding study demonstrated that the maternal average amount of intravenous fluids administered per millilitres per hour, positively correlated with infant maximum weight loss (Hirth et al, 2012).

All women having a caesarean section are given intravenous fluids. In postnatal wards where a lactation consultant is available, the baby can be monitored to ensure adequate nutritional intake and output when breastfeeding. Without the support of adequately trained staff, the recommendations from a review of the scientific literature concluded that, given the risk to the newborn associated with excessive weight loss, it is not prudent to incorporate maternal fluid intake into supplementation guidelines based on the existing evidence (Glasofer et al, 2022). Without leadership that values and supports breastfeeding and considers the harm of giving unnecessary commercial baby milk substitutes to the babies of mothers having intravenous fluids, nothing will change. Mothers have shown me photographs taken immediately post-caesarean section of their bloated babies at birth when having lost more weight than expected. Within a short time frame, because of the extra diuresis, the babies look normal. The same thing happens with the mothers and usually within several days the swelling disappears. On assessment, the parents will often say that the baby had two or three wet nappies within the first 24 hours. This is not normal output for a day-old baby and without time or a skilled person who can assess the baby, unnecessary commercial infant milk is likely to be given.

Lactation consultants

Currently, International Board-Certified Lactation Consultants (IBCLC) without an underlying qualification such as nursing or midwifery cannot be employed in maternity hospital postnatal wards in NSW, due to lack of recognition of the IBCLC qualification. The IBCLC is an international qualification that requires lactation consultant candidates to undertake studies in health sciences, such as human physiology, anatomy, infant and child growth and development, biochemistry and nutrition. Prior to sitting the International Board-Certified Lactation Examination (IBCLE), 90 hours of practical training and current lactation-specific education is required. The candidate may be required to complete between 300 and 1000 hours of supervised clinical experience, depending on previous education. While having a second qualification such as obstetrics or midwifery is advantageous initially, it is also a deterrent to maintaining the lactation qualification because updates are required every five years and maintaining a second degree is expensive and time consuming. No hospital in Australia employs standalone IBCLCs unless they have another degree and no university offers a standalone lactation course.

Without an employing an adequate number of lactation consultants to teach within the public hospitals breastfeeding knowledge is inadequate. Recently a very senior and experienced midwife who had returned to the postnatal coalface told me that after attending a lactation consultant run breastfeeding seminar for the first time in her career she felt competent and was able to latch and evaluate an effective breastfeed.

Some obstetricians and midwives have told me that they let the lactation qualification lapse due to cost and time, while others have left the lactation workforce because they no longer have the physical stamina for shift work or the need to maintain the mandatory education requirements for obstetrics or midwifery. Had they been employed as a lactation consultant without the tick-boxing requirements of the skills they are no longer using, their employment life as a lactation consultant may have been extended.

Qualified IBCLCs are a valuable resource used by midwives and doctors as minimal breastfeeding education is taught in Australian universities, including midwifery and medical courses where junior staff in public hospitals are expected to be taught on the job. Many academics designing the health courses within the universities have failed to recognise that the science of breastfeeding has moved on and either fail to recognise they do not know what they do not know or refuse to relinquish control. Australian breastfeeding rates are substandard, and in order to reach sustainable development gold targets breastfeeding knowledge needs to be disseminated through all education and health disciplines.

Birthing in public hospitals

In public hospitals, the majority of women are housed in shared rooms with shared bathrooms and toilets on postnatal wards, and are separated by curtains. During labour and birth in hospital, a delivery suite, operating theatre or recovery room provide an environment where a family member can remain to provide physical and emotional support to the mother. There the new mother receives multidisciplinary care depending on her needs. Following transfer to the postnatal ward, care of the mother and baby falls to a midwife, who in NSW public hospitals may have up to six mothers and babies allocated to her care.

In hospitals that have BFHI accreditation, step seven of the 10 steps to successful breastfeeding requires women to room in with their babies 24 hours a day, unless there is a medical reason not to do so. Rooming-in allows the mother to recognise infant feeding cues and to feed her baby when the baby is hungry. Without a single room, a family member cannot remain after visiting hours to help.

The shared rooms in public hospitals were not designed to house breastfeeding women with crying babies overnight, and research demonstrates that women do not like to be separated from strangers only by curtains. Curtains are not sufficient to make the women feel secure and are inadequate protections of a woman's privacy and confidentiality. They can be inadvertently opened and expose a mother to embarrassment when breastfeeding or pumping. The gender-specific nature of maternity care needs to be considered. Research from the United Kingdom and Australia indicates that there is a 100 per cent preference by women for single rooms with an en suite toilet and bathroom (Maben, 2009).

The Australasian Health Facility Guidelines (Australian Health Infrastructure Alliance, 2023) recommend single rooms in hospitals with a foldaway bed for a partner or family member to remain and provide support to the new mother. In an ethnographic study where women were interviewed about the postnatal ward environment, they gave the top score when asked about the importance of having a partner remain overnight to help (Scurry, 2021). New mothers said they needed the support of a partner or other family member, as often the midwives were busy and the mother could not care for the baby alone. Women who had a caesarean section said it was difficult to move due to the painful wound, a catheter and intravenous tubes, and without a family member present, it was unsafe.

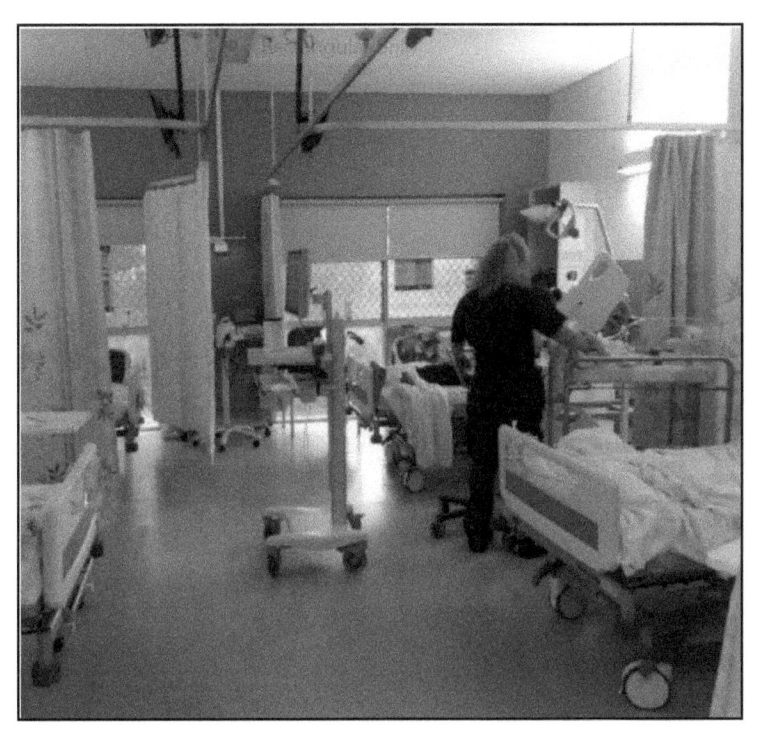

Shared four-bed ward with mothers and babies separated by curtains and rooming-in, 2021

Single rooms with foldout beds enable culturally appropriate care to be provided to Australia's multicultural and Indigenous population, where mothers receiving the support of female family members is normal practice. When I was in Alice Springs on a midwifery study tour, the charge nurse in the neonatal nursery told me Indigenous women expect to support their young mothers following birth, and there are 100 per cent exclusive breastfeeding rates of the hospital NICU infants because it is unsafe not to breastfeed within the communities. Single rooms also allow for a family member to remain, which helps to address the isolation and rural disadvantage of being a new mother when relocated to a central hospital service away from their own community.

Staffing allocation varies between states within Australia. Midwives and nurses have been campaigning in NSW to improve mother-and-baby staff ratios for many years. In the 1950s, when my brothers and I were born, and up until the 1970s when I had my first three children, women could remain in hospital for up to ten days, which gave mothers time to rest and recover from birth while learning to care for their babies. As the breasts changed during the first week and the milk increased, experienced midwives were able to guide the women. Now, new mothers have little time to rest and recover from birth before leaving hospital, and midwives spend a large amount of time admitting and discharging mothers and babies because the number of days has been stripped to the bare minimum (see Figure 4.3). Research from Queensland has demonstrated that neither public nor privately insured women are satisfied with postnatal care following birth in Australia, and the current service leaves most women ill-equipped and unsupported when having a baby (Zadoronjnyj et al, 2015).

Figure 4.3: Length of stay in days in NSW public and private hospitals following birth, 2007–2020. Source: Australian Institute of Health and Welfare, 2023

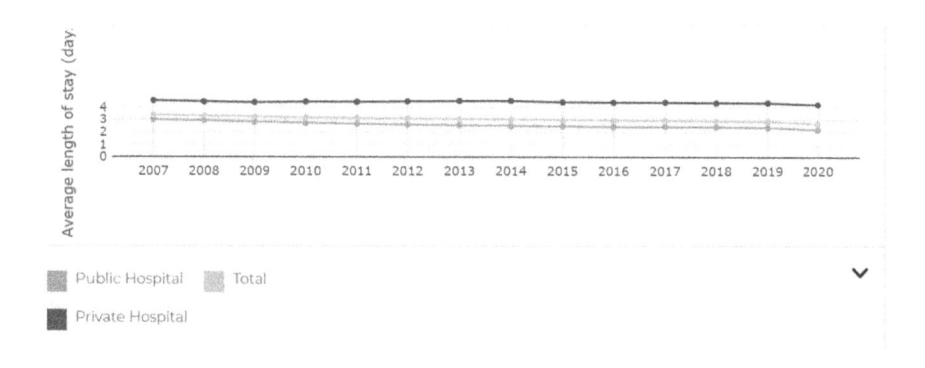

My story: Birth experiences

In 1976, when my second daughter was born, I remained for five days in a quiet country hospital postnatal ward with only three or four other mothers. I was given choice and midwifery support in the way I cared for my baby, whom I kept with me at the bedside most of the time. She was only returned to the nursery when I napped and was unable to watch her. She was exclusively breastfed and I was well supported by the midwives. Because I had a quiet, single room, my partner was free to come and go and the staff treated us as a family. I left hospital fully breastfeeding and confident.

In 1984, when my fifth child was born, the obstetrician in the large city hospital responsible for my care permitted me to go home four days after the birth. I pushed to leave because I was missing the other children. However, I soon regretted my decision, as I was tired and had the responsibility of four other young children in addition to the baby. My partner had little leave and soon returned to work. This baby did not return to her birth weight until she was a month old and was soon placed on complementary commercial infant milk due to slow weight gain.

In all five of my birth experiences, the institutions were in control, and I complied with the care regimes offered within the setting. I preferred the small country hospital environment, which allowed the midwives time to support me in a homely setting compared to the hustle and bustle of a big city university hospital. The five days of quiet allowed me to rest and recover while establishing breastfeeding, before going home to the demands of a new baby and toddler.

****

Improving postnatal care

In 2009, the then chief nurse and midwifery officer who led the Australian review into maternity services, Rosemary Bryant, stated there was a lack of an evidence base to guide health workers in the provision of early postnatal care. Furthermore, that it was crucial that new mothers be supported during the postnatal period (Commonwealth of Australia, 2009). With the continued increase in operative births and decline in breastfeeding rates, it appears a reassessment of postnatal care is long overdue.

Women who remain in hospital are more likely to be first-time mothers needing extra support and education while learning to breastfeed and care for their baby, or mothers with a baby in the neonatal nursery. Some women have underlying medical, surgical or obstetric complications requiring additional care. These women are at the highest risk of not breastfeeding or succumbing to mental health issues and require optimum postnatal care.

Often, infants can be slow to feed due to the type of birth, for example following a forceps or vacuum extraction (ventouse). Multiple birth babies, such as twins or triplets, can take a large amount of midwifery time because the infants are often small and require regular blood sugar level monitoring and more frequent feeding. To ensure adequate breastmilk, the mothers need help with feeding to make certain that they can hand express or pump to stimulate milk supply. Mothers of multiple babies have little time to rest. When staffing the postnatal wards, it is important such mothers are adequately supported. In NSW, where babies are not counted in staff-to-mother ratios, midwives are left with little time. If a mother has one twin in the NICU, and one with her in the postnatal ward, NICU is allocated funds to pay for the baby's care. However, on the postnatal ward, the cost of caring for the second twin is counted as one with the mother, who may have birthed by caesarean section and be unable to care for her infant by herself. Without a single room to allow a family member to remain and help, the mother and midwifery staff will struggle.

I had a midwife friend who resigned after a terrible night shift on the postnatal ward when a 17-year-old Indigenous mother dropped her baby in the middle of the night when she fell asleep. My friend told me she was attending another woman in the shared room behind the curtain and heard a strange sound, which she proceeded to investigate with a torch in the dark. She found the mother sitting up still asleep and her baby on the floor. Culturally appropriate care for an Indigenous mother is to have other women in the family helping. Because the young mother had complications, she had remained in hospital in a shared four-bed ward, with no accommodation to allow a family member to remain overnight. My friend picked up the baby and ran to the neonatal nursery, where the baby was cared for by the neonatal staff. My friend had to return to the busy ward. She was traumatised by the experience and asked me, 'What if I had not been in the room and heard the strange sound?' She resigned following that shift and now practises as a midwife in a small rural centre.

The high caesarean section rate renders many mothers unsafe to care for their infant alone. The anaesthetic takes time to wear off and painkillers make the mother drowsy, while the wound and compulsory postoperative in-dwelling urinary catheter and intravenous infusion hinder women's mobility. Current staff ratios of one midwife caring for up to six women and their infants are inadequate to support skin-to-skin contact safely on the postnatal ward, unless a family member is present and knows how to keep the baby safe.

Many maternity services operate outside the safe-sleeping guidelines, which state that you should never co-sleep or lie down holding a baby. Risk factors include:

- being over tired or unwell
- the parent or parents taking drugs that make them sleepy or less aware
- the baby is premature or small for their gestational age.

At the parliamentary inquiry into breastfeeding in 2007, women identified the four main concerns about breastfeeding during their hospital stay:

- overworked staff
- lack of skills in assisting with attachment difficulties
- inconsistent advice
- noise and embarrassment (Commonwealth of Australia, 2007).

Hospitals have failed to implement improvements to the postnatal hospital environment and increase staffing levels to enable safe sleeping arrangements, despite numerous recommendations.

Most women who remain in hospital are there because they are unwell or medicated and need help. Without providing a single room where a family member can remain to help care for the baby when having skin-to-skin contact or breastfeeding, the baby may not be safe. Babies are often brought to the staff work area to quieten the shared rooms during the night to allow the women to rest and keep the baby safe. This may not be optimum as the work area maybe left unattended when the staff are attending to other women and infants.

My story: Postnatal care done well

Having an inadequate number of single rooms during the COVID pandemic made infection control difficult in many shared postnatal wards because the required metre and a half separating women meant four-bed occupancy had to be cut.

During the COVID pandemic, my son and his partner were planning to have their first baby at the local birthing centre under the care of a midwife. The antenatal classes were attended online with Zoom. They attended Calmbirth classes, and the mother was healthy and well prepared for the birth. When the baby was due, the membranes ruptured spontaneously. However, the contractions were not regular or effective and nothing happened except the mother could not rest and got tired.

After nearly 24 hours, my son's partner was assessed at the hospital because of the risk of infection from the prolonged rupture of membranes. On ultrasound examination, the baby was in a breech position (bottom first). Without an experienced team, a breech birth is considered dangerous, and most breech babies are born by caesarean section.

My son asked for my opinion, as a caesarean section was not part of their birth plan. As there was no time to arrange another option, and with the lockdowns in place due to COVID, it would be difficult to organise an alternative. So I reluctantly agreed that they should go ahead as the doctors had recommended. The hospital was BFHI accredited, and the baby was placed in skin-to-skin contact with the mother while on the operating table and in the recovery room, where they had to remain for some time due to anaesthetic complications. My son was able to stay with his partner and baby throughout the surgery and recovery, as well as during the hospital stay, as a single room with a foldout bed was provided. They remained on the postnatal ward for three nights and four days, when they were discharged home under the care of the birth centre midwife due to a shortage of hospital beds.

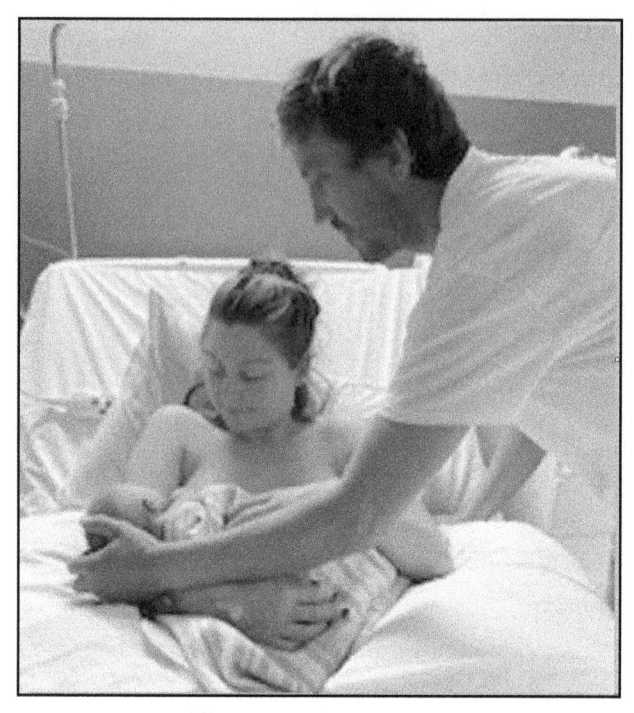

*New parents following an emergency caesarean section
for an undiagnosed breech presentation*

My son provided all the nappy changing and infant soothing, while his partner breastfed and rested for around a month at home. I provided lactation support, while the other grandmother and sister stayed to help. The baby never needed commercial baby milk, and he continued to breastfeed beyond the age of two. Like many couples, my son and his partner are unlikely to have another baby because the physical and emotional price on the mother of having surgery followed by two or three years of unpaid work is too high.

Breastfeeding and cultural variations

In 2021, the *Australia's Mothers and Babies Report* stated 34 per cent of mothers were born overseas. As shown in Figure 4.4, the most common countries of birth were India (5.4 per cent), New Zealand (2.6 per cent) and the United Kingdom (2.5 per cent).

Breastfeeding varies from culture to culture, and during times of political upheaval. There are many myths surrounding colostrum, which may be discarded because it is considered 'dirty'. For some migrant mothers, bottle-feeding may be a sign of socio-economic status, or a necessity if they have to get back to work. There are women who expect to be supported by other women. In some South Asian societies, women other than the mother breastfeed or give pre-lacteal feeds to the infant rather than colostrum. For many new mothers, not being able to have a female family member stay with them and help them in hospital does not meet their cultural needs.

Figure 4.4: Ten most common maternal countries of birth, 2021. Source: Australian Institute of Health and Welfare, 2023

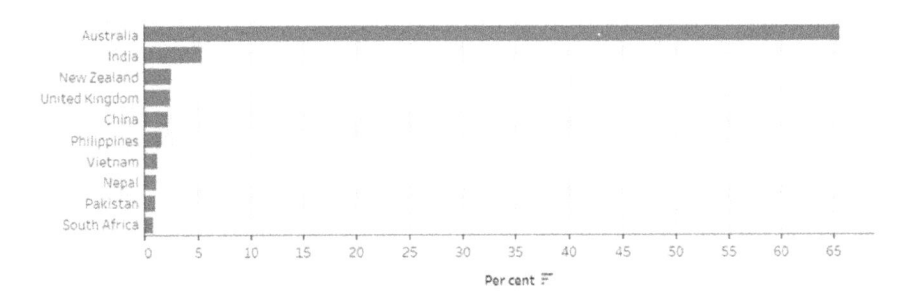

My story: The importance of cultural understanding

I have provided breastfeeding care for many migrant women. Within our local community we have a high proportion of Chinese women. One mother I was asked to see had a profound effect on me and the way I administered her care. At the consultation her mother was there tidying the cubicle, and I noticed she had brought in homemade chicken soup. When I examined the new mother, I found she had extremely engorged breasts and the baby could not latch. When trying to assist with hand expressing, I could see the new mother was extremely stressed and the milk would not flow. In an attempt to relax her, I asked questions about the baby's grandmother and if the baby was a first grandchild. The new mother told me her mother had flown from China to help her following the birth and, yes, her baby was the first grandchild. She also told me that when she had been born her parents were considered enemies of Mao and had been sent to work in the fields. They had almost starved during the Cultural Revolution while she had been raised by her grandparents.

While we were talking the infant started to cry and needed feeding. As the grandmother could not speak English, I asked the new mother to translate what I was saying for her mother. When trying to hand the baby to the grandmother earlier I had realised she was frightened. My heart broke, as she wanted to help her daughter but did not know how. I followed my instincts and placed the baby on my chest next to my heart and demonstrated how I rocked my grandchildren when they were unsettled, gently explaining to the grandmother that I would sing and dance. Placing the infant at the grandmother's chest and showing her how to keep the baby close to her heart, I guided her into a swaying motion and hummed 'Sylvie', an old Harry Belafonte favourite my grandbabies loved. We two grandmothers gently danced together holding the baby between us, and then the baby's grandmother started to hum 'Sylvie' with me. While we danced with the baby, I saw the grandmother beam a smile at her daughter. And, as I turned, I also saw that the milk dribbled from the new mother's breasts as she wept.

Another mother I was asked to see had a 10-year-old daughter born in China who she had been unable to breastfeed. When consulting with the woman following the birth of her son, I realised that the baby boy was not sucking and just sleeping at the breast. It was Easter and the woman wanted to go home as her husband had holidays and they wanted to be together. I explained the baby was not getting any milk and demonstrated to both parents how to express by hand. I also demonstrated how to set up and use the electric pump. After several cycles of the suction rhythms, a pink nipple that had never seen the light of day was pulled from the dark areola. The woman had inverted nipples, which had not been recognised and, just as his sister before him, the baby boy could not attach. Because the couple had gone home after my consultation, I was anxious about the baby's fluid intake and followed up the parent's progress with the home maternity nurse the following day. She laughed and said the baby was feeding hungrily and getting lots of milk and the parents were just so happy it had been a pleasure for her to visit.

Daisy was another young woman I cared for. She was from Nigeria and was far from her family when she had her baby by caesarean section. The staff told me she was depressed and having difficulties latching and breastfeeding her baby. During the consultation, I realised Daisy was homesick and wanted her mother. We talked about her family and what her mother would tell her. I supported Daisy to breastfeed her baby, demonstrating with a doll and knitted breast, talking about the importance of skin-to-skin contact when she was able. The consultation took considerable time, but when I left I was satisfied I had helped Daisy. The following day, when I looked in, Daisy told me she had spoken with her mother by mobile phone in Nigeria the previous evening, and her mother had told her she must breastfeed her baby, as it was important for good health. Daisy went on to exclusively breastfeed. Breastfeeding is not solitary. It requires time, knowledge, compassion and kindness.

****

Supporting women and providing choice

In Australia and overseas, there is considerable evidence that supports the benefits of a vaginal birth after caesarean section (VBAC) for women. However, currently the incentives for public and private institutions and doctors support repeat caesarean section. A larger remuneration is paid for performing the operation, as well as offering the convenience of scheduling operative births to suit hospital and medical schedules compared to a normal vaginal birth. There is also the issue of litigation. If something goes wrong, it is difficult to defend the decision not to perform a caesarean section in an individual case. However, on a population basis it is women who bear the physical and emotional cost of having to care for a newborn following their abdomen being cut open.

In Australia, although not mandated, it is recommended that following a caesarean section, women do not drive for six weeks. In NSW, there are limited options for women to receive specialist breastfeeding home visits. When I conducted an audit into breastfeeding services at our hospital, one woman wrote, 'I can barely get out of my pyjamas, let alone come to the breastfeeding clinic. It would be helpful if a lactation consultant could come to me'. Without a Medicare rebate for lactation consultants, only women in some private health insurance funds or of a higher socio-economic bracket can afford lactation support at home, and currently there are an inadequate number of lactation consultants to support women in the community.

There are many programs, such as one-on-one care with a known health professional, that support better outcomes for birthing women. Breech clinics can assist in the use of external cephalic version (ECV), a procedure performed by a skilled professional, often using ultrasound, to reduce the need for a caesarean section. Continuity of one-on-one midwifery care is beneficial for both normal healthy women and women with high-risk pregnancy issues. In the Northern Territory, a program to have an Indigenous doula accompany Indigenous mothers from outlying islands to centralised hospitals is being trialled. For many women, distance and rural disadvantage may deny them access to programs that support normal birth, as hospitals may not have the resources.

5

The Baby-Friendly Hospital Initiative

The BFHI is an evidence-based education program designed to achieve the World Health Assembly's maternal, infant and young child nutritional targets. The design and implementation of the BFHI is a tool aimed at improving breastfeeding rates at international, national and local levels. Introduced into Australia in 1992 by UNICEF/WHO, the initiative changed its name to the Baby-Friendly Health Initiative to include community, neonatal and paediatric care of infants. BFHI is currently managed by the Australian College of Midwives.

The Australian Government has a responsibility to support BFHI because Australia is a signatory to the UN's human rights agreements and also because most Australian women birth within taxpayer-funded hospitals. The current breastfeeding rates throughout Australia are well below international benchmark, and a multisector approach is required if they are to improve.

Why is BFHI important?

The BFHI is an integral component in the provision of high-quality care to mothers and babies. Health workers are pivotal in educating mothers and, as most infants are born within the hospital setting, health workers are ethically obliged to do no harm. While breastmilk is natural, breastfeeding is a learned skill. *The Best Start: report on the inquiry into the benefits of breastfeeding* published in 2007, states:

> Even though it is a natural act, breastfeeding is also a learned behaviour. Virtually all mothers can breastfeed provided they have adequate information, and support within their families and communities and from the health care system. They should also have access to skilled practical help from trained health workers, lay and peer counsellors, and formally certified lactation consultants, who can help to build mothers' confidence, improve feeding technique, and prevent or resolve problems (Commonwealth of Australia, 2007).

When teaching new parents, health professionals and people within the community about breastfeeding, I will ask if they can learn to dance or play tennis in one lesson. Breastfeeding needs to be learned and the myth suggesting otherwise is harmful to women. On a breastfeeding education day at the Taronga Park Zoo, the educators explained to the participants that humans, like their nearest mammalian relatives (for example, chimpanzees or great apes) learn from other mothers. The zoo educators told us of a female gorilla who had been raised in captivity at the zoo and was artificially inseminated as part of a breeding program. Following much anticipation, excitement and expense, the birth finally came. The new mother gorilla discarded her infant, as she did not know what to do with it, and the baby gorilla died. The mother gorilla had no role models to teach her and she did not know how to be a mother.

At the WHO country coordinators' meetings of industrialised nations for the BFHI, the importance of the BFHI in meeting the six infant nutritional targets for infants under five in the

SDGs – as discussed in Chapter 2 – was emphasised. To achieve BFHI accreditation, hospitals need to adhere to the 'the ten steps to successful breastfeeding' (see Figure 5.1) and maintain the standards set down by the accreditation guidelines, including adherence to the WHO's International Code of Marketing of Breastmilk Substitutes. Hospitals are assessed every three years. During the COVID pandemic in Australia, assessments were conducted online and not face-to-face.

Figure 5.1: The WHO/UNICEF BFHI's Ten Steps to Successful Breastfeeding

Critical management procedures	
1a	Comply fully with the International Code of Marketing of Breastmilk Substitutes and relevant World Health Assembly resolutions.
1b	Have a written infant feeding policy that is routinely communicated to staff and parents.
1c	Establish ongoing monitoring and data-management systems.
2	Ensure that staff have sufficient knowledge, competence and skills to support breastfeeding.
Key clinical practices	
3	Discuss the importance and management of breastfeeding with pregnant women and their families.
4	Facilitate immediate and uninterrupted skin-to-skin contact and support mothers to initiate breastfeeding as soon as possible after birth.
5	Support mothers to initiate and maintain breastfeeding and manage common difficulties.
6	Do not provide breastfed newborns any food or fluids other than breastmilk, unless medically indicated.

7	Enable mothers and their infants to remain together and to practise rooming-in 24 hours a day.
8	Support mothers to recognise and respond to their infants' cues for feeding.
9	Counsel mothers on the use and risks of feeding bottles, teats and pacifiers.
10	Coordinate discharge so that parents and their infants have timely access to ongoing support.

(WHO, 2018)

The ten steps to successful breastfeeding require all group one staff — that is, clinicians who have direct patient contact with breastfeeding mothers and infants — to have 20 hours of breastfeeding education to learn 16 core competencies:

1. How to teach mothers to hand express.
2. How to discuss infant feeding in the antenatal period of pregnancy.
3. Care and use of nipple shields.
4. Nipple variables.
5. Breast engorgement and breastfeeding or expressing.
6. Treatment of mastitis.
7. Strategies to increase breastmilk supply.
8. How to store and transport breastmilk at home.
9. Techniques for expressing breastmilk postnatally.
10. How to prepare infant formula per NHMRC guidelines.
11. How to give parents information about artificially feeding.
12. How to clean and sterilise feeding equipment.
13. Techniques for suppression of lactation.
14. Management of a healthy term sleepy baby in the first twenty-four hours.
15. Care of a late preterm and/or low birth weight infant.
16. Dummies usage.

(Australian College of Midwives, 2018)

My story: BFHI-accredited hospitals in NSW

In 2000, I moved to NSW from Victoria, where I had worked only in BFHI-accredited facilities. I discovered three hospitals in NSW were BFHI accredited, including the Royal Hospital for Women in Randwick where I initially worked. When I moved to Newcastle I worked in a public hospital and was rostered to work in a postnatal ward night nursery. Babies were separated from their mothers overnight and housed in the nursery. They were cared for by nurses and midwives, who woke the mothers when the babies were ready to feed. The babies were often supplemented with expressed breastmilk or commercial baby milk by night nursery staff to let the mothers rest.

I saw conditions that I had rarely seen in BFHI-accredited hospitals, such as mothers with engorged breasts. Babies in BFHI hospitals room in with their mothers and can feed when the infant shows hunger signs, which helps to prevent breast engorgement. Bonding and confidence in caring for the baby is enhanced when mothers and infants remain together. The mother learns to recognise their infant's feeding cues and can feed the infant when hungry. Rooming-in and responsive feeding by the mother aids in increasing breastmilk hormones and breastmilk production, thereby reducing the need for supplementation with commercial milk.

Mothers or parents who have their infants cared for in a nursery overnight may have unrealistic expectations of a normal infant's behaviour because they have not cared for an infant overnight. The most common call I received when on night duty in an emergency department of a large maternity hospital was from exhausted parents who did not know how to stop their infants crying following hospital discharge.

The hospital was a teaching facility attached to a university, and hospital managers were receiving reports from the university educators that student midwives were dissatisfied with breastfeeding education because it was inconsistent and not evidence based.

BFHI was a natural fit as an evidence-based program. Newcastle's population was changing, with midwives from other states arriving and advocating for BFHI, so the local sub-branch of the Australian College of Midwives (ACM) held a workshop at the local league's club. BFHI had aroused political controversy within some areas of the hospital sector. However, more than 50 participants from different hospitals throughout the district attended and, in 2007, the John Hunter Hospital became the fourth hospital in NSW to be accredited (and the first within NSW within a decade).

****

Breastfeeding rates in Australia

In Australia across and within different states and territories, there is evidence of a wide disparity in exclusive breastfeeding rates.

Figure 5.2: Proportion of infants aged 0–3 years by exclusive breastfeeding status for at least 6 months state and territory, 2021–2022. Source: Australian Institute of Health and Welfare

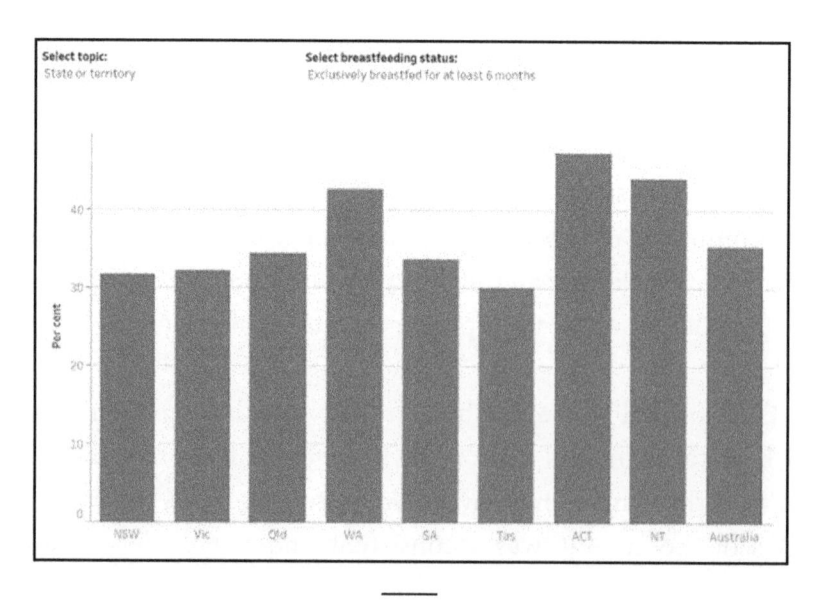

While all states and territories are below the SDG targets for 2030, which aims to have at least 50 per cent of infants exclusively breastfed at around six months, some places do better than others (see Figure 5.2). The Australian Bureau of Statistics (ABS) website states two in five infants were exclusively breastfed to around 6 months of age in 2022.

The obvious question is why does this disparity exist? Are the reasons socio-economic factors or differences among ethnic/cultural groups, types of postnatal environments, BFHI status of hospitals within the area, breastfeeding support skills, the workload of the midwives, length of postnatal hospital stay, community support measures or other unknown factors? These probable reasons are yet to be adequately synthesised and understood by Government agencies, health providers, community members and breastfeeding mothers. The disparities at hospital discharge within NSW range from 84.1 per cent in Northern NSW, down to 59 per cent in South Western Sydney (see Figure 5.3).

Figure 5.3: Infant feeding at discharge from hospital by Local Health District, full breastfeeding, 2019. Source: NSW Government, 2020

Local Health Districts	Number	Per cent
Sydney	5,277	69.7
South Western Sydney	8,372	59.0
South Eastern Sydney	7,784	75.2
Illawarra Shoalhaven	3,392	75.0
Western Sydney	10,488	69.2
Nepean Blue Mountains	3,420	67.7
Northern Sydney	7,077	73.3
Central Coast	2,935	78.0
Hunter New England	7,902	74.8
Northern NSW	2,213	84.1
Mid North Coast	1,768	78.8
Southern NSW	1,160	81.2
Murrumbidgee	1,752	73.8
Western NSW	2,555	73.1
Far West	157	72.7
Other, not stated	1,006	73.3
All LHDs	67,258	71.1

Although lower socio-economic status or level of education achieved are listed as reasons for low breastfeeding outcomes, in NSW breastfeeding rates at hospital discharge in the private hospital sector, where women are better resourced and from a socio-demographic group that can afford to pay health insurance, are currently less at hospital discharge when compared to the public sector. In 2023, in NSW, no private hospitals were BFHI accredited, and unless women are admitted to private beds within BFHI-accredited public hospital postnatal wards, privately insured women do not receive the benefit of BFHI.

Figure 5.4: Breastfeeding rates in private/public hospital system, NSW 2007–2022. Source: NSW Government, 2022

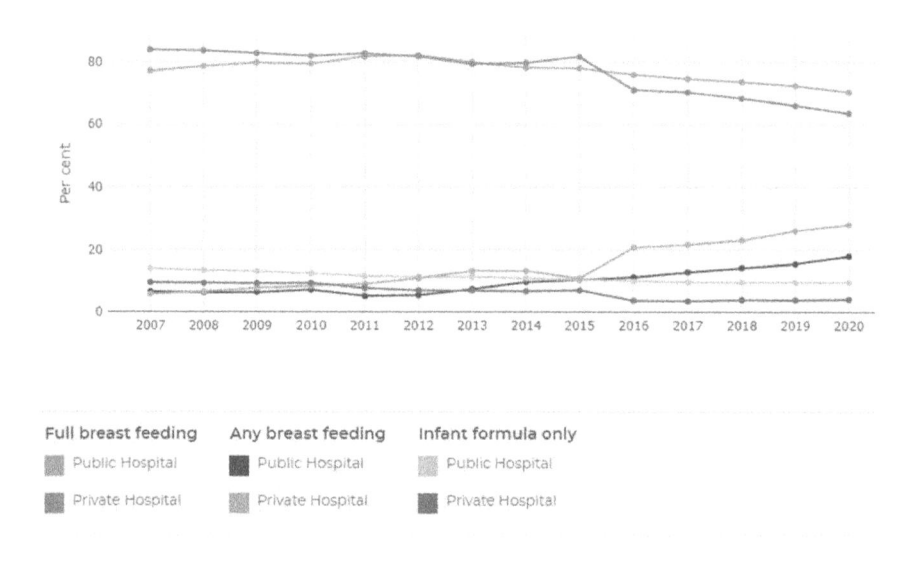

Prior to BFHI being reinvigorated in NSW in 2007 and six more hospitals BFHI accredited, private hospitals had higher breastfeeding rates at hospital discharge compared to the public sector. This may have been because of the improved accommodation and longer hospital stay for privately insured women where women may remain in a single room with a family member overnight or stay longer to rest and recover from birth, with extra time to establish breastfeeding and learn mothering skills. However, as more public hospitals became BFHI accredited, things began to change. In 2016, the public hospital breastfeeding rates at hospital discharge surpassed those from the private sector. In 2023, the public hospital state average at hospital discharge in NSW was 72.4 per cent of infants fully breastfeeding, surpassing the privately insured sector, which was at 66 per cent. Figure 5.4 compares full breastfeeding, mixed feeding with commercial infant milk and breastfeeding, or full commercial baby milk feeding within the public and private hospital system in NSW at patient discharge between the years of 2007 and 2022.

Nothing but breastmilk

Step six of the ten steps to successful breastfeeding states, 'Do not provide newborns any food or fluids other than breastmilk unless medically indicated'.

While any breastfeeding rates (including combined breastfeeding and commercial baby milk feeds) are higher in the private sector (31.1 per cent compared to 19.8 per cent in 2022), research demonstrates that the longer-term impacts of introducing commercial baby milk are that exclusive breastfeeding duration rates decrease in the short and long term. Unless the mother expresses breastmilk to maintain her breastfeeding hormone levels, the hormone levels drop. The empty breast is a trigger to make more milk. Because commercial baby milk takes a longer period for the baby to digest, the baby takes longer between feeds, which reduces the amount of the time the infant is at the breast and inhibits the breastfeeding milk production. I often tell mothers about my colleague breastfeeding her triplets. She told me she sat in a chair and fed and fed while her family fed her. Within the private hospital sector women are cared for by private obstetricians and paediatricians, many of whom lack day-to-day breastfeeding knowledge and defer to the midwives for lactation support. Without implementing the BFHI or employing an adequate number of lactation consultants or midwives with breastfeeding skills and education, mothers may not receive correct breastfeeding information and commercial baby milk may be given to their baby.

My story: Successful breastfeeding in practice

Recently a health worker sought me out for lactation support during her planned elective caesarean in a private hospital. She explained her family had ongoing psychological issues from a previous traumatic caesarean birth, resulting in the baby undergoing care for some time in a neonatal intensive care unit. She wanted lactation consultant advocacy and support, knowing she would be tired and in pain following the birth. Due to the COVID pandemic, I was not permitted to visit the mother in hospital. However, we prepared during the pregnancy for what was to come and frequently communicated via text messaging.

The mother hand-expressed from 35 weeks gestation after seeking her doctor's permission and had a small amount of frozen breastmilk to use in hospital if necessary. She arranged with the obstetrician to have the baby placed in immediate skin-to-skin contact in the operating theatre or with her husband if she was incapacitated for any reason. The baby's first feed occurred following the birth while having skin-to-skin contact in the recovery room.

Because the mother had developed sore nipples with the previous child, education on correct positioning and attachment had been discussed during the antenatal period, and video resources were provided prior to the birth. The mother took a copy of the Australian Breastfeeding Association elimination chart into hospital, and we discussed what normal output for a breastfeeding baby was, including urates, which are orange-type crystals passed in the wet nappy, and when this was normal.

When the mother was back in the postnatal ward following the birth we were in contact via text when required. Together, we organised for her to initiate breast stimulation for 10 to 15 minutes on each breast with the electric breast pump every three to four hours if the baby would not suck. She was aware that, as the colostrum was thick, the electric pump was for stimulation only and she needed to hand express to obtain colostrum to feed the baby. She used a three-minute video from the UK BFHI parent resources video site, which she had placed in her 'favourites' during the antenatal period on the mobile phone (http://www.unicef.org.uk/babyfriendly/baby-friendly-resources/video/hand-expression/).

This video is short and easily understood and demonstrates how to hand express. The baby vomited and gagged mucus for the first 24 hours following the caesarean section, which is normal. Both parents had received antenatal education as to expected changes in weight in an infant receiving intravenous fluid (IV) administration during a caesarean section. These infants often lose more weight than infants born without the administration of IV fluids, so when the infant had lost 11 per cent of birthweight on day five they were not surprised. The mother told me she was bemused when the midwife instructed her to give a 90-millilitre bottle of commercial baby milk prior to hospital discharge as her own milk, which had initially been delayed, was now coming in in abundance. The mother had the confidence to not use the commercial baby milk and breastfeed. At two weeks of age, the little girl was thriving and continued to be breastfed to WHO recommendations.

****

6

The Neo-Baby Friendly Hospital Initiative

The Convention on the Rights of the Child (1989), article 9, states:

> Parties shall ensure that a child shall not be separated from his or her parents against their will, except when competent authorities subject to judicial review determine, in accordance with applicable law and procedures, that such separation is necessary for the best interests of the child. Such determination may be necessary in a particular case such as one involving abuse or neglect of the child by the parents, or one where the parents are living separately and a decision must be made as to the child's place of residence.

Maternal-neonate separation after birth is standard practice in modern neonatal care of sick or premature infants. While around 70 public hospitals are BFHI-accredited in Australia and skin-to-skin following birth within the first hour is normal practice for healthy term infants, Australia's most vulnerable and at-risk premature infants are separated from their mothers and remain in incubators in neonatal care units.

The importance of Neo-BFHI

Nils Bergman, a South African specialist whose primary professional interest is the study of kangaroo mother care (KMC) believes that separation of the infant and mother is harmful (Bergman et al, 2010). KMC is an intervention aimed at improving the outcomes among preterm and low birth weight newborns, and is defined by the WHO as prolonged skin-to skin contact between the mother and infant. Although the definition of KMC is not clearly defined, the evidence shows there are many benefits such as reducing the risk of death, hypothermia, severe illness, nosocomial infection (hospital acquired infection) for stable premature infants or babies under 2 kilograms (Chan et al, 2016).

Recent scientific discoveries such as the development of the infant microbiome, epigenetics and neuroimaging have provided scientific explanations that were not available in the past. Advances in technology demonstrate the advantages of KMC and skin-to-skin contact compared to incubator care, which can hamper the emotional and social development of the infant and result in neurologic maladaptation to our actual environment (Bergman et al, 2004). KMC is normal for the newborn infant and improves physiological stability and breastfeeding outcomes. When a baby remains in skin-to-skin contact, they do not release the stress hormones caused by separation. When educating parents, I often explain how crying and stress impacts infant breathing, use up calories and may deplete an infant's energy (Bystrova et al, 2014). When babies are in skin-to-skin contact and breastfed, they establish a nutritive sucking breathing pattern, remain warm, gain weight, have a better quality of sleep and improved sleep cycles, which help with brain maturity.

Globally, around 15 million infants are born prematurely every year. Historically, preterm and sick infants admitted to neonatal wards have been subjected to policies and practices that do not support (and are barriers to) successful breastfeeding (Moore et al).

In Australia, there are no BFHI-accredited neonatal nurseries. Due to the history of separation of mothers and infants in neonatal care, the ongoing silos have created a divide, which is inconsistent and confusing for staff and families.

Most premature and sick newborns in Australian hospitals are treated in neonatal intensive care units (NICUs) by specialist doctors (neonatologists) and neonatal nurses. Australian neonatal units have been slow to adopt neo-BFHI principles, and parents remain visitors to the nursery, as they are seen as separate from the infant. While the maternity ward midwives may be encouraging the mother to express her breasts frequently to build up a supply of breastmilk to sustain her infant, the neonatal staff may be telling her to go back to bed and have a good night's rest while they supplement the infant with commercial baby milk. When parents are asked annually in the NSW Health Public Hospital Survey if they received conflicting advice, they repeatedly say they were given inconsistent breastfeeding information. On the postnatal ward in my role as a lactation consultant, I have spent many hours every week transitioning the mother and baby back to breastfeeding because infants have been tube or bottle fed in the NICU and cannot breastfeed.

Modification of Ten Steps to Successful Breastfeeding

Kirsten Nyquist studied and worked with premature infants, demonstrating the three guiding principles of neo-BFHI and how they were implemented in the hospital where she worked. I attended conferences in 2011 and 2015 in Uppsala, Sweden to hear Nyquist speak about the implementation and how the neo-BFHI group modified the BFHI's ten steps to successful breastfeeding for the neonatal nursery worldwide (see Figure 6.1).

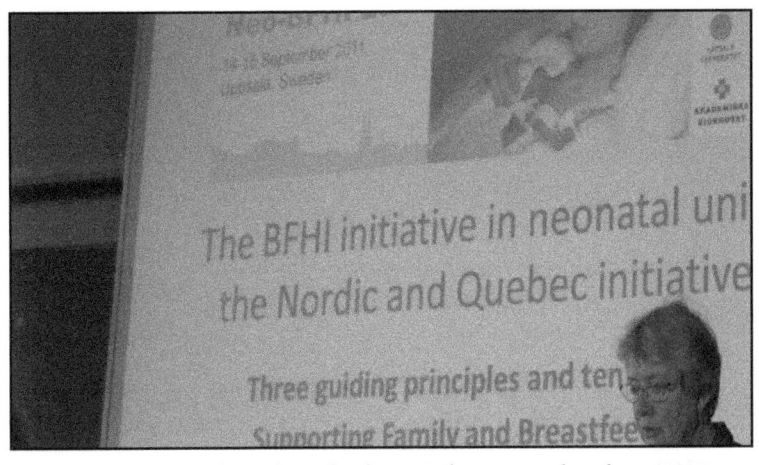

Kirsten Nyquist launching the three guiding principles of neo-BFHI at the Neo-BFHI Conference, Uppsala, Sweden, 2011

The three guiding principles of neo-BFHI are:

1. Staff attitudes towards the mother must focus on the individual mother and her situation.
2. The facility must provide family-centred care supported by the environment.
3. The health care system must ensure continuity of care from pregnancy to after the infant's discharge.

Neonatal BFHI steps to successful breastfeeding

1. Have a written breastfeeding policy, adapted to infants who require neonatal care that is routinely communicated to all concerned staff and to parents.
2. Treat every mother with sensitivity, empathy and respect for her maternal role. Support her in taking informed decisions about milk production and breastfeeding according to her own wishes.
3. Educate and train all staff in specific knowledge and skills necessary to implement this policy.

4. Inform all pregnant women about initiation of lactation in the event that the infant is born premature or ill.
5. Encourage early and continuous and prolonged skin-to-skin contact (kangaroo mother care) without unwarranted restrictions, and offer opportunities for mothers to remain with their infants 24 hours a day.
6. Inform, encourage and support mothers in early initiation and establishment of breastfeeding and maintenance of milk production.
7. Encourage and support mothers in early initiation of breastfeeding, with infant stability as the only criterion. Give mothers individual support.
8. Give the mother's own milk as first choice, and pasteurised donor breast milk as second choice, fortified when indicated.
9. Encourage breastfeeding on demand as early as possible, with semi-demand breastfeeding as transitional strategy for preterm infants (the mother nurses when an infant shows signs of interest, and in addition offers her infant the breast in order to reach a breastfeeding frequency per 24 hours that is sufficient for adequate infant milk intake)
10. Offer the infant a pacifier for relief of pain, stress and anxiety, and for stimulating the uptake of nutrients during tube-feeding. Introduce bottle-feeding when there is a reason.
11. Provide a family-centred and supportive physical environment.
12. Support the father's presence without restrictions, as the mother's main supporter and the infant's caregiver.
13. Plan the infant's discharge by early transfer of the infant's care in the neonatal unit to the parents. Inform the mother about where she can obtain breastfeeding support after discharge by staff or members of breastfeeding support groups with adequate knowledge (Haiak et al, 2015).

Figure 6.1: Guiding principles of Neo-BFHI and three of the Ten Steps to Successful Breastfeeding. Source: Kirsten Nyquist, 2011

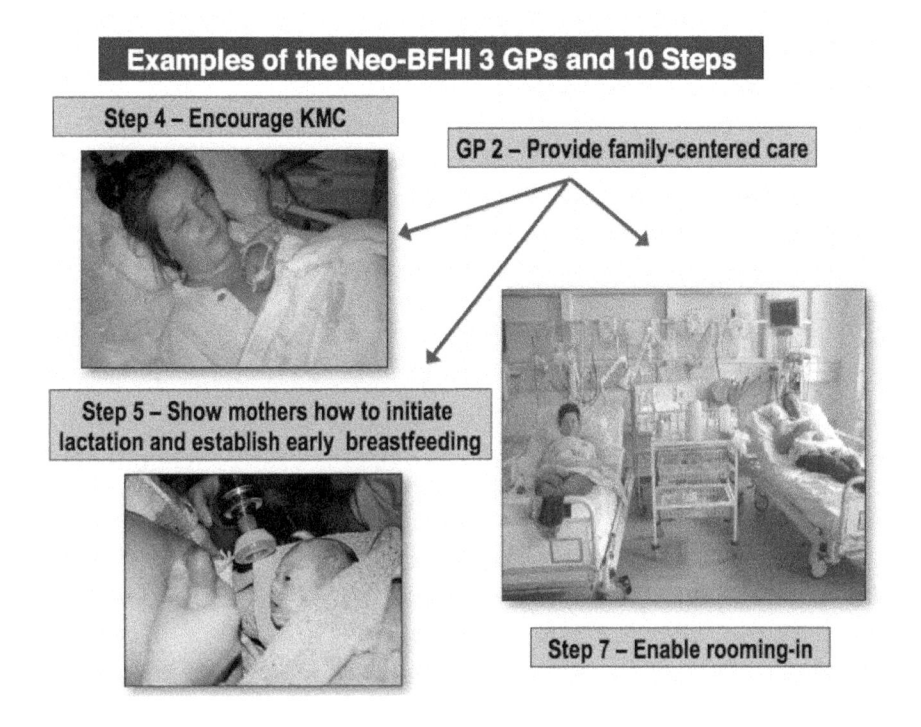

In 2017, a cross-sectional survey of 917 neonatal units globally aimed to measure compliance with the three guiding principles and neo-BFHI's expanded ten steps to successful breastfeeding. The study found in 917 neonatal wards that the median international overall score was 77 from 100. Guiding Principle 1 (respect for mothers), Step 5 (breastfeeding initiation and support) and Step 6 (human milk use) had the highest scores — 100, 88 and 88 respectively. Step 3 (antenatal information) and Step 7 (rooming-in) had the lowest scores, 63 and 67 respectively. High-income countries had significantly higher scores for Guiding Principle 2 (family-centred care), Step 4 (skin-to-skin contact) and Step 5 (breastfeeding initiation and support).

The authors concluded that the high number of participating units indicated international readiness to expand baby-friendly standards to neonatal settings and recommended hospitals and governments should increase their efforts to better support breastfeeding in neonatal wards (see Figure 6.2).

My story: Giving confidence

On one occasion, a mother on the postnatal ward whom I had tried to see all day telephoned me from NICU. The mother invited me to come to NICU as she was hoping her son would have a breastfeed when she was having her first cuddle. In Australia, many health professionals believe neonates do not get their sucking reflex until abound 36 or 37 weeks. In Sweden, Kirsten Nyquist told us that there is no such thing as non-nutritional sucking and when keeping mothers and infants together in skin-to-skin contact infants breastfeed sooner.

'Ollie' was four days old and premature. He weighed 1700 grams and was being assisted to breathe in an isolette, fed by a nasogastric tube and had a lot of equipment attached to his body.

When I arrived, the mother showed me a 50-millilitre bottle of her milk which was being fed to Ollie by nasogastric tube, but because her breasts were so hard and full I encouraged her to soften them by expressing before Ollie came to her. She pumped for about five minutes, and there was a lot of milk all over her breasts by the time we took off the pumping kit and said to the nurse we were ready for Ollie.

He was lifted from the isolette to his mother's knee with many wires and tubes. As Ollie got close to his mother his little arms started to tremble with anticipation and when he was placed near a breast he started to lick off the spilt milk. He tried but was unable to latch onto the nipple because the nipple was too big or his mouth too small. I asked for a small nipple shield, which I coated and filled with expressed breastmilk and placed onto the mother's nipple. She then gently drew him onto the shield holding him close. He began to make little sucking motions and soon got into a sucking and breathing rhythm. The mother's nipples were leaking milk into the shield and I was dripping expressed milk onto the shield near Ollie's mouth. Ollie continued to make little butterfly-wing sucking motions with his cheeks and was drawing in the milk while the mother cooed encouraging sounds to her son. The interaction between the mother and baby took around 20 minutes and then the little boy fell back from the breasts asleep and relaxed. His mother was overjoyed.

The NICU nurse asked me how much milk she should give Ollie down the nasogastric tube after she had returned him to the isolette. This was difficult to answer as it is hard to estimate what goes in and these babies are so little and tire easily so I suggested about half the required quota. I came away on such a high as I knew I had given the mother confidence in her own abilities.

****

Pain and neonates

Researchers have demonstrated repeated painful procedures can be stressful for young infants and cause long-term neurological damage (Harrison, 2017). In the past, it was assumed infants did not feel pain and because of risks such as respiratory depression, pain relief was not prescribed. In 2016, The American Academy of Paediatrics said, 'preventing or minimizing pain in neonates should be the goal of paediatricians and other health professionals because it is ethical but also because repeated painful exposures have the potential for deleterious consequences'. The Academy added that, 'non-nutritive sucking, provision of breastfeeding or providing expressed human milk, or skin to skin contact have been shown to be useful in decreasing pain scores during short-term mild to moderately painful procedures and should be consistently used'.

I have a friend whose second child was born at 26 weeks gestation, and is one of the youngest surviving premature infants born within a Victorian hospital from that time. My friend told me she did not think her daughter would survive, and that she was afraid to visit her in the NICU because the baby would stop breathing when the nurses took her from the incubator to hold. My friend said she thought the baby associated being taken from the incubator with another painful event. In neo-BFHI-accredited nurseries, infants and parents can have skin-to-skin contact 24/7, with procedures being performed while they have that contact.

Skin-to-skin contact or breastfeeding has been demonstrated to reduce infant's pain when having painful procedures. During World Breastfeeding week in 2023, Professor Denise Harrison from Melbourne University's School of Nursing presented research locally to health professionals on the advantages of skin-to-skin contact and breastfeeding when performing painful procedures on preterm infants.

Human milk banks

Many researchers have demonstrated the benefits of a mother's own milk when a baby is premature or unwell (Neu, 2014). In 2016, researchers recommended efforts be made to support the production or the use of mother's own breastmilk. They demonstrated that among extremely low birth weight infants, not being fed human milk increased the risk of developing necrotising enterocolitis (NEC) (Parker et al, 2021). NEC is a disease seen primarily in preterm infants, with risks including extremely high morbidity and mortality, as well as cost to the healthcare system. The long-term complications include strictures and adhesions of the intestine, cholestasis, short bowel syndrome, failure to thrive and neurodevelopmental delay. In 2020, a research study strongly encouraged human milk intake in the early days following birth and demonstrated the association between less neonatal infection, NEC and death (Ochoa et al, 2020).

In NSW, it took many years of lobbying by consumers and breastfeeding advocates before a human milk bank was set up in Sydney by the Australian Red Cross. Some neonatal nurseries were unwilling to accept other mothers' freely donated unpasteurised milk due to the risk of infection or contamination. A lactation consultant and paediatrician who was involved in setting up a human milk bank told participants at the Lactation Consultants of Australia and New Zealand conference in Canberra in 2014 that the red tape and wrangling when deciding if breastmilk was a food or a 'therapeutic good' held up the establishment of a donor milk bank for years at the hospital where she was employed.

One Sydney neonatal nursery commenced using medically prescribed pasteurised donor milk when the neonatal nursery was donated pasteurising equipment by parents of premature twins because there was no state-run donor milk bank.

The lack of inclusion of women in the way infants are fed has led to a quiet movement of civil disobedience due to a disagreement over priorities between the providers of infant care and some mothers. For some women, the rules surrounding donor milk are so tedious that they do not divulge they are milk sharing, which can be problematic. While it is fine to give donor milk in most cases, premature infants are vulnerable due to their gestational age and there are risks.

The Red Cross human milk bank, like the blood bank, accepts free donations of human breastmilk from lactating mothers. The donor milk is screened, pasteurised and sold. The current cost is around AU$900 a litre. In neonatal nurseries, donor milk is limited to very premature infants due to the cost. Unfortunately not only does this send the wrong message to mothers, but in the long term it may also be false economics when weighed up against the health benefits to mothers and infants and the impact of the dairy industry on the environment.

My story: Positive results with donor milk

I was contacted by a lactation consultant who had been chastised by management because she had acquired some donor milk for a premature baby in a rural hospital. The baby was 34 weeks gestation and not tolerating the commercial baby milk feeds. The mother was so stressed due to the pressure of a sick baby and demands by the nursery staff for breastmilk that the lactation consultant organised donor milk from Sydney. Once the donor milk arrived and the pressure was taken off the mother, she started to produce enough milk of her own and the donor milk was not used. The lactation consultant had another mother with supply issues and wanted to use the untouched pasteurised milk for the second woman. The milk was within date and unopened; however, the red tape involved was too cumbersome and the milk was not used.

****

Breastmilk substitutes and the Australian National Breastfeeding Strategy

BFHI and neo-BFHI must comply with the International Code of Marketing Breastmilk Substitutes and relevant World Health Assembly resolutions to maintain accreditation. When I came to NSW in 2000, the commercial baby milk manufacturers were gold sponsors at health events and influenced policy makers at many levels. With the implementation of the NSW Breastfeeding Policy there has been some change. However, the lack of government leadership and multidisciplinary input within BFHI has meant neo-BFHI within Australia has not progressed. Neonatal units and their staff continue to receive education and kickbacks from commercial baby milk companies, and makers of bottles and teats, which leads to misinformation being given to staff, and undermines new mothers and breastfeeding supporters.

The Australian National Breastfeeding Strategy recognises babies admitted to the neonatal intensive care unit are at a higher risk of not being breastfed compared to healthy babies. Breastmilk is important for premature infants because the milk produced in the first few days following birth contains high concentrations of antibodies to help the infant fight infection and is more easily digested than commercial baby milk. There is strong evidence, as well as many government documents and reports, which details the dangers to vulnerable premature or sick infants who are not breastfed (Smith et al, 2018). So it is surprising the recommendations – including that neonatal units be BFHI-accredited – in the National Breastfeeding Strategy 2019 and Beyond have not been implemented. I can only surmise that the power of the baby milk manufacturers is too great and their influence permeates management decisions.

Figure 6.2: An example of a free non-WHO Code compliant education event held by the local public children's hospital supported by Nestle, Mum and Me

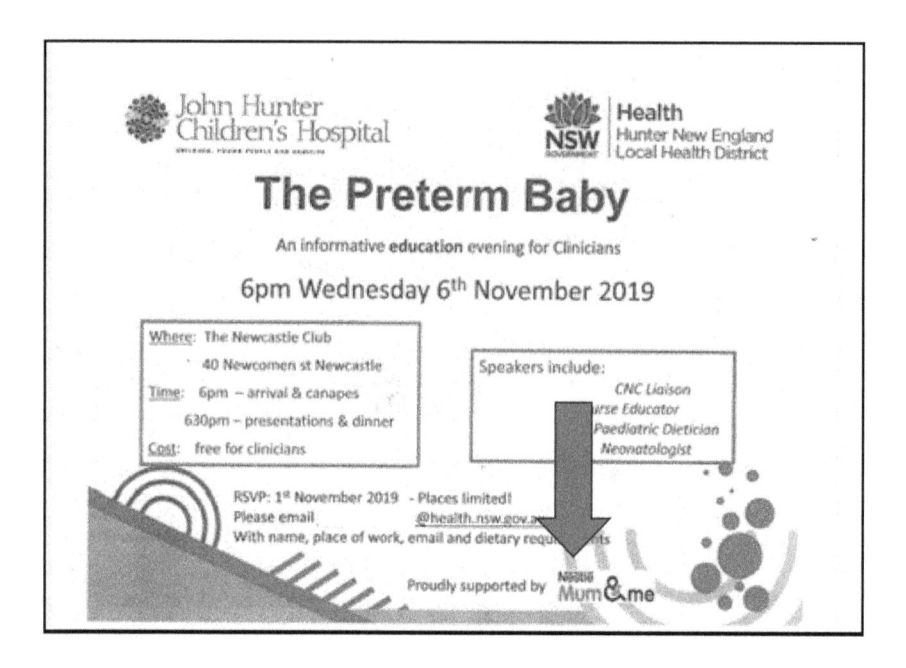

My story: Lactation support for NICU babies

While working in a postnatal ward, I received a referral for a mother with a baby in the neonatal unit. The baby had been admitted to the neonatal nursery at 37 weeks gestation due to breathing problems. I attempted to see the mother in the postnatal ward three times before going to the neonatal nursery to seek her out. She was lying in a large armchair with her baby on her chest having skin-to-skin contact for the first time. While the baby remained connected to breathing apparatus, both mother and infant appeared content as the infant's father looked on. After I'd introduced myself, the mother told me she had asked to see a lactation consultant as none were available in the NICU and she had many questions. Although she and her husband were medical doctors and knew breastmilk was optimum, they had little practical knowledge. They needed advice on how to achieve an adequate daily breastmilk supply to feed their baby.

While the general nurse caring for their baby listened, I delivered the basics, and when I finished they reaffirmed what was required and requested a follow-up consultation. When I saw the mother some days later, although her baby was much improved and gaining weight, her confidence had been undermined while the baby was in NICU. Transitioning from having a baby with breathing difficulties to a well baby was hard for her, and she was extremely anxious.

I frequently provided care for babies returning to the postnatal ward from the neonatal nursery where the infants have either been tube or bottle-fed. These mothers and babies require intensive lactation support if a baby is to be returned to breastfeeding. In a research study in which I was involved between 2021 and 2023 (in production), it was demonstrated that the babies admitted to the neonatal nursery were fed more commercial baby milk and had poorer breastfeeding outcomes than babies receiving standard care. The women in the study were motivated to breastfeed and provided with one-on-one lactation support. However, because the baby was admitted to the neonatal unit and under the care of NICU staff, breastfeeding outcomes were reduced when compared to women whose babies were not in NICU. In my opinion, the lack of breastfeeding success in NICU is because of lack of confidence by staff when supporting the women to breastfeed and the ease of bottle and tube feeding without having to need to negotiate with parents.

The women told me they felt stressed when separated from their baby. Research demonstrates that by keeping mothers and infants together in a BFHI-accredited neonatal nursery, infants are discharged home from hospital sooner because parents are partners in the nursery care of their infant and gain confidence when rooming-in (Silva et al, 2022; Maastrup et al, 2022).

****

Breastfeeding support for NICU and sick infants

Premature infants take more time to learn to suck because of their gestational age, while sick infants may be too unwell because of an infection or too sleepy due to jaundice to suck. These babies and mothers require additional breastfeeding support. In the Boston Medical Centre in the USA, the neonatal nursery employs mothers who have had a previous premature baby within the nursery to support current mothers of premature infants. These women provide empathy and physical support while educating the new mothers in useful ways to help their infant.

Breastmilk not only improves the outcomes of sick or premature infants but also shortens hospital stays, thus reducing the economic burden on institutions in the short and long term. I am often asked by parents on the postnatal ward to accompany them to the neonatal unit to help with breastfeeding because they cannot find lactation support there. By adopting neo-BFHI, the neonatal unit would become more family friendly, educate staff with the knowledge to address the breastfeeding needs of mothers and provide best outcomes for babies within their care. Children's hospitals throughout Australia, when compared to other areas of health, are very well resourced and receive generous funding from the public through events such as the Good Friday Appeal. When sick children in institutions are used to raise money, there is a need for transparency and consumer input to ensure that parents' and community expectations are being met.

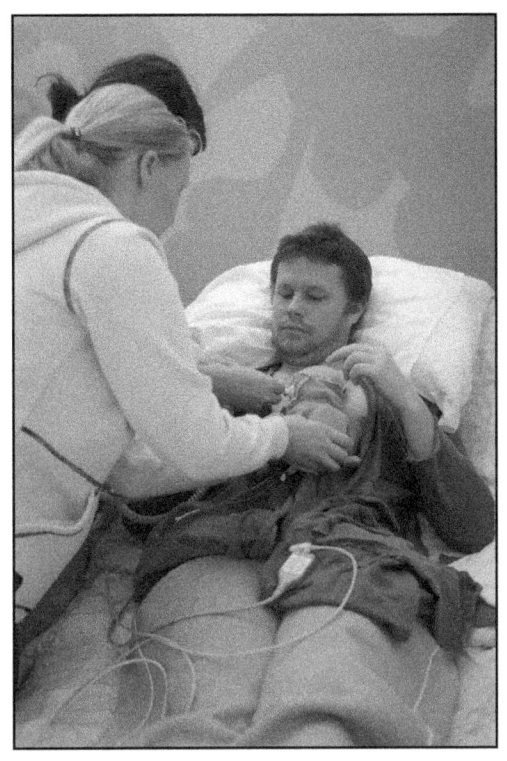

Parent of a premature infant living in at the Neonatal Intensive Care Unit at the Uppsala hospital. Living within the neonatal unit, while providing skin-to-skin contact with their baby 24/7, promotes bonding, parental confidence and increased breastfeeding outcomes.

My story: Parents disempowered

Consider two quotes from mothers interviewed in Kirsten Nyquist's research. One of the women said, 'You need this little extra empathy, somebody who says, "You are doing great"'. Another mother stated, 'I felt summoned, just like some kind of feeding machine; that was my task, not cuddling'.

I recently had coffee with the mother of my granddaughter's 11-year-old classmate from primary school. The mother told me she was still angry about how she had been treated when her daughter was admitted to a neonatal unit. She said she had been made to feel like an outsider and was not included in her daughter's care during the long neonatal intensive care stay. She said the staff had bonded with her daughter, even giving her a pet name. When her daughter was medically fit to go home, the staff had dressed the baby in special clothes for hospital discharge. The mother said that although she was grateful to the competent staff, her lack of inclusion in her daughter's care had made her feel inadequate, scared and ill-prepared as a mother. While she did not appreciate the graduation ceremony marking her baby's discharge, she did not speak up at the time because she did not want to jeopardise her daughter's care.

Since birthing practices were institutionalised in Australia and throughout my lifetime, partners have been disempowered by exclusion from birthing and postnatal practices that, in turn, have impacted bonding. Lack of bonding is a risk factor for both maternal and paternal maltreatment of an infant. In a 2018 research study of 1008 couples in Japan, intimate partner violence at one month postpartum was found to be associated with a lack of mother-to-infant affection and bonding, and associated with a lack of father-to-infant bonding (Nishigori et al, 2020).

Physical barriers such as incubators and other types of equipment can prevent parents from becoming involved (Garnica-Torres et al, 2023). Many fathers tell me they feel unwelcome in the NICU; that the tubes and monitoring equipment make them afraid to touch their baby. There is considerable research that indicates that fathers have a strong influence on a mother's breastfeeding decisions and experiences (Vetcho, 2022; Mörelius et al, 2021). Emerging neuroscience validates the importance of immediate skin-to-skin contact and breastfeeding following birth and during the early postpartum period, due to the interaction of differing hormones that drive protective parental behaviours. Hence every effort needs to be made to keep parents and infants together to facilitate parent and infant bonding within all areas of the hospital system. Publicly funded neonatal nurseries within Australia have an obligation to practise evidence-based best practice and for physicians to do no harm.

Supporting successful breastfeeding

In 2007, the parliamentary inquiry into breastfeeding made three recommendations to the Australian Government that were not implemented and remain relevant today:

- Recommendation 14. 'That the Department of Health and Ageing fund the Australian College of Midwives to run the Baby Friendly Hospital Initiative in Australia, to facilitate the accreditation of all maternity hospitals'.
- Recommendation 15. 'That the Department of Health and Ageing work with the Australian Council on Healthcare Standards (and/or equivalent accreditation organisation) towards including Baby Friendly Hospital status as part of the accreditation process'.
- Recommendation 16. 'That the Commonwealth Government, when negotiating future Australian Health Care Agreements, require state and territory governments to report on the number of maternity wards in public hospitals that have been accredited under the Baby Friendly Hospital Initiative' (Commonwealth of Australia, 2007).

In Australia, in 2024, 21.4 per cent of 276 birthing facilities are BFHI accredited. The ACM continues to manage the BFHI, with 59 accredited facilities Australia-wide. The individual numbers of BFHI facilities are listed by states and territories on the ACM's website. Due to the COVID pandemic, the number of accredited facilities had fallen from 70 in 2021 as the increased workload in providing data for the on-line accreditation team shifted to already overworked hospital staff on the ground, rather than the accreditation team which prior to COVID visited on site. This is a remarkable achievement without Australian Government resourcing, which had been recommended by the parliamentary inquiry. BFHI is supported across Australia through the contributions of volunteer breastfeeding advocates, ACM member subscriptions and the cost of the BFHI facility assessment.

The Office for Women seems ideally suited to oversee and manage BFHI. It is not optimum that the ACM be left to roll out a discipline that requires other areas of health input given that midwives only provide care for infants during the postpartum period. The WHO and the Australian National Health and Medical Research Council (NHMRC) recommends exclusive breastfeeding for six months, and then continued breastfeeding combined with complementary family foods for 12 to 24 months, or as long as the mother and baby may desire. Midwives do not have authority within the differing disciplines within health, and a new approach is required to include neonatal, community and paediatric care to better support new families and improve breastfeeding outcomes.

7

A History of Infant Feeding

Since the beginning of time, it has been known that breastfeeding passes on special properties from the mother to the child. In Greek mythology, Zeus placed his son Heracles on the breast of Hera, his sleeping wife, so that Heracles would receive godlike attributes from Hera. Heracles' birth mother, unlike Hera, was a mortal. When Hera awoke to find an unknown infant feeding from her breasts the milk ejected into the night sky as she pushed the infant away. The squirting milk drops provided the ancient Greeks with an explanation of the Milky Way.

Pharaoh's daughter found Moses a wet nurse after finding him floating in the Nile, as she knew he would die without a mother's milk. The evolution of infant feeding has been well documented over the centuries, and it has always been known that, if the mother could not feed her own infant for any reason, wet nursing from another human mother was best. Wet nursing was a respected profession until it was replaced by the production of commercial baby milk.

An Egyptian obstetrician told me breastmilk sharing was common in his culture and that 'milk siblings' cannot marry. Did the Egyptians have knowledge as to the epigenetic properties of breastmilk? The Qur'an explains that a child nursed from another women's breast becomes a relative of the nursing women, and other children who share the same mother's milk are not to marry under Islamic law.

Researchers in Turkey have hypothesised that infants wet-nursed on a regular basis may share similar epigenotypes, and if the epigenetic modifications can be inherited in the next generation, marriages between individuals breastfed by the same woman may have similar consequences as consanguineous partnerships.

Historically in Europe and the United Kingdom, wet nursing was common in the upper classes. It was important that noble families produced an heir, and aristocratic women often had their children cared for by other women and wet-nursed. When women moved into the cities from rural areas during the Industrial Revolution, working-class mothers had to employ women to feed their children.

In Central Australia, many Indigenous people did not come into contact with white Australia until the 1930s. Since then, literacy and numeracy skills have remained low. Until time has evolved to allow education of subsequent generations, the Indigenous population is at risk of great harm due to lack of scientific knowledge. When I was touring the Northern Territory with Indigenous midwives, they spoke of their frustration during the COVID pandemic because some isolated First Nations people were listening to the teachings of fundamentalist Christians on the internet and refusing to have the COVID vaccine. Breastfeeding remains the safest way to feed a baby and fortunately new Indigenous mothers are supported by their communities to breastfeed.

My story: Wet-nursing in PNG

When I was nursing in PNG in 1977 and 1978, breastfeeding and wet nursing was a natural everyday event and what women did. It is normal for the 'big man' within a village in PNG to have more than one wife. A bride price is paid to the family of the woman in goods of value, such as pigs, shells and cassowary feathers, to recompense the family for the loss of their daughter.

At the Kimbe hospital, following the death of a first wife in childbirth, I witnessed the second wife take on the breastfeeding responsibilities of the dead mother's newborn, while breastfeeding her own infant. The mother had died giving birth to her seventh daughter following a postpartum haemorrhage complicated by anaemia. Anaemia is common in PNG, due to malaria and hookworm. During the grieving period and because the baby was another girl (the big man now had 14 daughters), the baby was left at the hospital for several days and wet-nursed by other lactating mothers. As I was breastfeeding at this time, I too would breastfeed the little girl when I heard her cry. Wet nursing is the safest option in the tropics.

When my family come to visit I found out from them that Miti, our babysitter, was wet-nursing my own daughter. I would rush home with full breasts to find Jessie ambivalent about being fed by me. I had noticed Miti's little boy, who was around 2 years of age, clinging to his mother and not happy that he was being supplanted by another child, but I had not realised Jessie was sharing his milk.

****

Wet-nursing rules and superstitions

Seventeenth-century French obstetrician, Jacques Guillemeau, did not like auburn-haired wet nurses because it was assumed they had a hot temper. He believed that this was harmful for the breastmilk. Guillemeau favoured the natural mother breastfeeding her infant and listed the disadvantages of wet nursing in his writings *The Nursing of Children*:

- The child may be switched, with another put in its place.
- The affection between the child and the mother may diminish.
- A bad condition may be inherited by the child.

- The nurse may transmit an imperfection of her own body to the child that could then be transmitted to the parents (Guillemeau, 1612).

An eighteenth-century view

In the United Kingdom in 1748, Oxford-educated physician Doctor William Cadogan came to prominence after writing 'an essay upon nursing and the management of children from birth to three years of age'. The letter was written to the governors of a foundling hospital and discredited the swaddling of infants.

Doctor Cadogan was scathing of women and nurses who fed newborn infants rich pre-lacteal feeds that were common amongst wealthy women, who thought they were a good idea at that time. Pre-lacteal feeds can be any food given prior to the onset of lactogenesis two. In the eighteenth century bacteria were not understood, and the butter or pigs' fat that was used as a pre-lacteal food may have been contaminated, was certainly unnecessary and make the baby sick.

When treating diarrhoeal illnesses in infants, Doctor Cadogan prescribed three- to four-hour spacing between feeds to rest the infant's gut, thus restricting breastfeeding. In the case of exclusively overfed breastfed infants, this would have helped alleviate the watery stools and pain from too much milk.

Doctor Cadogan did not distinguish between breastmilk and complementary foods, which may have been contaminated and caused the diarrhoea. Rather than cut out the complementary foods and only breastfeed, he regulated breastfeeding and recommended babies be fed every three to four hours. He placed no time restrictions on the length of feeds but forbad breastfeeding overnight, which would have caused the breastfeeding hormone levels and production of the mother's own milk to drop. Doctor Cadogan had no scientific basis for his ideas, but his strong personality and reputation brought about changes to the way women breastfed and were taken up by other medical men.

Undertaking research into Doctor Cadogan, I found an article entitled 'William Cadogan, 18th Century Physician' (Short, 1960). Short reported that Cadogan may have plagiarised his ideas some 20 years earlier from a dissertation for a degree by Doctor Conyers, a physician at the Foundling Hospital. In a letter from the same period, an unnamed colleague who had recently fathered a child wanted to introduce the new practices of less restrictive clothing at home. He asked the matron about practices in the Foundling Hospital as reported by Doctor Cadogan and the governors and recorded her reply:

> You may imagine I was a little surprised to find she seemed puzzled at my question and told me she knew of no alteration from their former method; that the dress which I desired to see was the same as it had always been. ... I am at a loss to reconcile this part of (the governors') conduct viz. to recommend any scheme to the public of which they have not made trial themselves ...

The author then became quite heated. He concluded:

> I was greatly disappointed, expecting to have rally'd my wife out of half at least of her child's clothing, whilst she on the contrary turn'd the tables on me and cried out, ay, ay, my dear. How like the men, they are fond of novelty, thought it a pritty thing, talked of it, recommended it and then thought no more of it. I fancy, Sir, a committee of women would not be useless there and offer it to your and their consideration, for I

verily believe, Sir, our great grandmothers were very good nurses and very good housewives.

The influence of Truby King

Sir Truby King was another physician with a forceful personality. His medical training began in Edinburgh, and his training was in mental health. He had no children of his own but adopted an ideology that supported raising children on a schedule, with specific times for feeding, sleeping, bathing and toileting. After qualifying as a doctor and marrying Isabella, he was appointed as medical superintendent of Seacliff Lunatic Asylum in 1889, on the South Island of New Zealand. King turned the asylum into a productive farm, where he promoted fresh air, exercise, good diet, work and recreation as the appropriate treatments for inmates with mental illness. King was interested in the link between nutrition and diet as a preventative cause of insanity. When on a study tour to Japan, King was impressed by the physical fitness of the Japanese and noted the custom of prolonged breastfeeding by Japanese women.

At the farm, the death rate of bucket-fed calves was 20 per cent. As teenagers we raised bucket-fed male calves and sold them at market when grown. Without their mother's milk the calves were prone to diarrhoea or death when fed powdered buttermilk, either due to lack of cleanliness in the teats, tubing and buckets, or contaminated milk powder as a result of poor storage conditions. Were the high death rates of calves on Doctor King's farm caused by lack of cleanliness in the feeding equipment or contaminated milk products?

King and his wife Isabella had no children of their own. Following the adoption of their child who was failing to thrive, at his wife's request King turned his attention to developing an alternative modified form of cow's milk for babies. Rather than promote the birth mother to breastfeed more often, King's methods of feeding schedules down regulated breastfeeding hormones and reduced a mother's milk supply, thereby creating a need for breastmilk substitutes that he had encouraged dairy companies to make. King's methods were widely advocated in Australia.

He adopted an ideology that supported raising children on a schedule, with specific times for feeding, sleeping, bathing and toileting. Some described King's methods of childcare as turning infants into 'little machines', although they did reflect the ideas of the English upper class at that time.

King trained Karitane nurses (Karitane was King's home on New Zealand's South Island) to teach mothers to care for their babies, promoting domestic hygiene and his scheduled feeding methods. While the promotion of hygiene may have saved the lives of infants, the scheduling of infant feeding downregulated the breastfeeding hormones and the mother's own milk supply.

My Aunt Alice was trained as a Karitane nurse in New Zealand and achieved her triple certificate (general nursing, midwifery and Karitane nursing), a source of great pride for our grandmother.

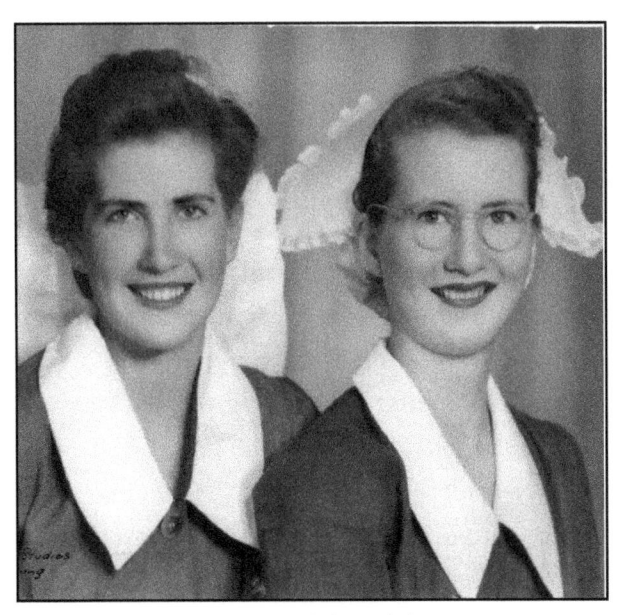

Karitane nurse, Alice Coddington (left) with her sister Bonnie (c.1940s)

While King disapproved of women being educated, he used influential women such as Lady Victoria Plunket, the wife of the New Zealand Governor General, to promote his 'scientific principles'. Lady Plunket, an aristocrat whose godmother was Queen Victoria, was also the mother of eight children and believed in the benefits of creating a professional nursing service to support mothers and babies. She travelled widely with King and promoted Karitane nursing.

In 1908, Lady Plunket said, 'Up to now, mothers have been left to untangle for themselves the great difficulties of rearing their babies, and over and over again little ones have had to suffer through want of knowledge as to the best food to give them under their changing circumstances. All mothers, rich and poor, should have the benefit and supervision of a women who is specially trained and fully qualified to help mothers' (Plunket, 1908).

King's wife supported his work in a widely read newspaper column entitled 'Our Babies'. In 1924, his book *Feeding and Care of Baby* was published and marketed throughout the English colonies. King thought parents should not pander to infants and that infants should be left to cry it out. Cuddling was considered spoiling, and he recommended infants be cuddled at a regular time each day for no longer than 10 minutes. He believed, without routine, babies become 'unproductive and self-indulgent adults'.

Following the First World War, King's ideas were promoted throughout the English colonies. In some parts of Canada, such as British Columbia, health professionals and childcare advisors counselled parents to adopt the new, regimented scientific mothering baby care routines recommended by Luther Emmett Holt, an American paediatrician, and Truby King.

Luther Emmett Holt came to prominence by improving hygiene standards in cow's milk products sold in the tenements of New York. Like King, Holt promoted the idea of regimented and disciplined parenting. In 1894, he published *The Care and Feeding of Children: A Catechism for the Use of Mothers and Children's Nurses*, which included the following advice. 'Babies under six months should never be played with and the less of it at any time the better for the infant. They are made nervous and irritable, sleep badly, and suffer from indigestion'.

Scientific mothering

In Australia, the physicians who promoted 'scientific mothering' and laid the basis for the subsequent care of women and babies in hospitals came from an elitist patriarchal system. They had little respect for woman and a lack of understanding of breastfeeding. The theories of Doctors Codagan and King had been developed as a result of working with motherless children or working with motherless calves and cow's milk. The English patriarchal class system, which denied woman an education, did not have the benefits of scientific knowledge in the early nineteenth century when promoting the use of breastmilk substitutes, and many of the myths created during that time persist today.

Physicians were part of an imperialist system that required women to produce babies to become tools to grow the economy and wealth of Britain. Rather than help women and infants to breastfeed, the physicians reflected the views of the times and the elite. Infants became ill and in many cases died after being fed unnecessary breastmilk substitutes, such as contaminated pre-lacteal feeds or contaminated cow's milk. Physicians failed to promote structural reforms, such as lactation breaks for women required to work in the factories of the Industrial Revolution, supported the separation of mothers and infants, and promoted ideologies of timed feeding and allowing infants to cry it out.

By limiting an infant's time at the breast, they also created a need for breastmilk substitutes. Scientific mothering was well suited to the emerging hierarchical hospital system, and the regimented practices of military nurses and nuns who cared for postnatal women and did not have the practical experience of independent midwives or breastfeeding women.

Figure 7.1: Mothers fully breastfeeding at three and six months, Victoria, 1950–1992. Source: Australian Institute of Health and Welfare

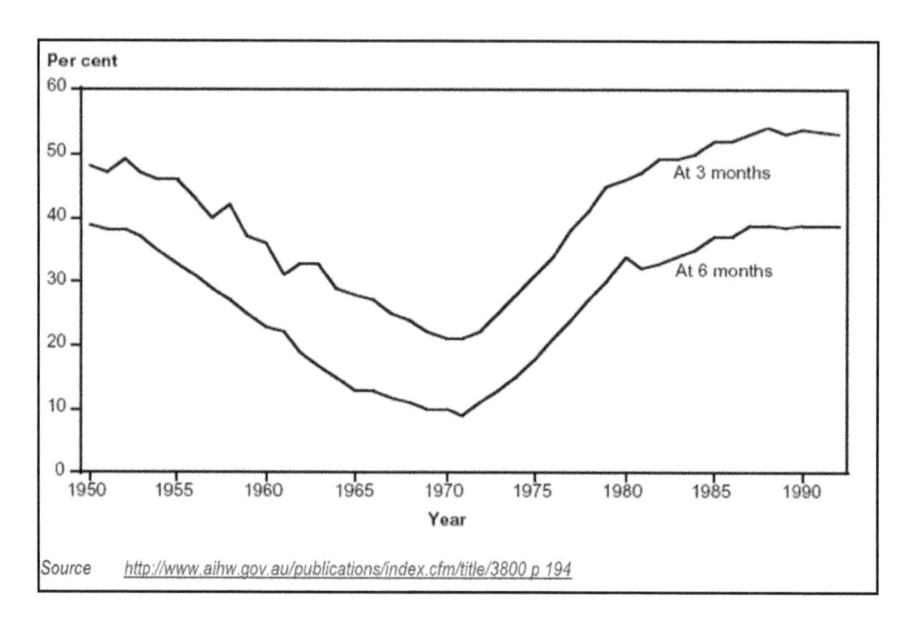

[Figure 7.1: Line graph showing percentage of mothers fully breastfeeding at 3 months and at 6 months in Victoria from 1950 to 1992. Both curves decline from 1950 to a low point around 1970, then rise again through the 1980s. Source: http://www.aihw.gov.au/publications/index.cfm/title/3800 p 194]

When I had my children and throughout my midwifery career, I found that many of the heads of obstetric services were bullies who used their positions to subjugate others and pursue their own interests. These professors had no interest in helping women breastfeed and left the practicalities to the midwives who had been trained within the hospital obstetrical service and had little authority. Figure 7.1 shows that breastfeeding rates for 3-month and 6-month-old infants in Victoria in the 1970s were at an all-time low.

Arvo Henrik Ylppo

At the same time as Doctor King was promoting his ideologies in Britain and the colonies, Arvo Henrik Ylppo (1887–1990) set up a public health system in Finland in 1922 (Dunn, 2007). As a Finnish paediatrician, he significantly improved Finnish maternal and infant mortality and morbidity figures. Ylppo was a kind man from humble beginnings, the fifth of 12 children from a farming family in central Finland. He became a paediatrician because he had seen his mother's anxiety when his siblings became ill.

Ylppo had practical experience of prematurity in infants as he studied them throughout his long life, bringing about positive change in paediatrics. He was curious and travelled widely to study different cultures and their medical problems, and was often seen dropper feeding premature babies for hours. At the time of his death in 1992, infant mortality rates had changed from 10 per cent in 1920 to 0.6 per cent in Finland. Yippo disliked the practice of fasting premature infants, which was recommended by two Boston paediatricians and used in the 1950s to prevent vomiting and oedema. In 1954, in response to this practice, Ylppo wrote a letter to the paediatric community.

> Both vomiting and edema which are the starting points for this hunger therapy are ambiguous phenomena attributable in their etiology to very many reasons. I do not consider them sufficiently justified premises for such a radical method of feeding as 2–4 days complete fast. I feel further that many premature infants continuously supplied during the fetal period with both food and plenty of water and growing rapidly must suffer in a special manner from a complete break in administration of fluid and food ... vomiting and edema cannot be prevented by

complete fast; indeed on the basis of all that has been said I am of the opinion that we must try to arrange to feed the premature infant immediately after birth in conformity with nature and the conditions of the fetal period.

Ylppo is revered in Finland as a result of the contribution he made to the lives of Finnish people.

Obstacles to breastfeeding

In the past, most women were taught to breastfeed by their mothers, other women, female family members and independent midwives. Many current new mothers do not have this benefit. When my third baby was born, because he was a big baby and wanted to feed often, my mother encouraged me to introduce a dummy. Giving the dummy resulted in an inadequate milk supply because he sucked on the dummy rather than stimulating my breasts and breastfeeding hormones by more frequent feeding. I know she was trying to help but her lack of correct knowledge undermined the amount of milk I was able to produce.

In *A History of the Australian Breastfeeding Association*, authors Jill Barnard and Karen Twigg (2014) relate that some general practitioners in the 1940s were concerned by the dangers of not breastfeeding, as many babies contracted 'summer diarrhoea'. As the scientific mothering movement spread and babies were weaned those living in poor social conditions without money for safe feeding alternatives many babies died. In a report from Wonthaggi, a mining town in Victoria where meticulous records were kept at the infant welfare centre during the Great Depression the link between poverty and the importance of continued breastfeeding was illustrated. Ten babies died following weaning because families lived in circumstances described by the nurse as bad. They did not have money to buy appropriate substitute milk, the facilities to sterilise bottles and teats and make up substitute baby milk, or money for medical support (Smith, 1993).

My husband's great uncle died at age three from summer diarrhoea in 1924 probably due to a lack of adequate refrigeration in which to store cow's milk which caused long term grief to the family. My nephew was saved at four months of age after contracting summer diarrhoea. He was administered intravenous fluids in hospital after being fed with either contaminated bottles, teats or commercial baby milk during a very hot February in NSW.

8

The Unique Qualities of Breastmilk

In 2016, in *The Lancet*'s breastfeeding series, Keith Hansen wrote, 'If breastfeeding did not already exist, someone who invented it today would deserve a dual Nobel Prize in medicine and economics. For while 'breast is best' for lifelong health, it is also excellent economics. Breastfeeding is a child's first inoculation against death, disease and poverty, but also their most enduring investment in physical, cognitive, and social capacity' (Hansen, 2016). In the same series, it was estimated that the lives of 823,000 children and 20,000 mothers could be saved from getting breast cancer worldwide each year through universal breastfeeding, together with an estimated US$300 billion worth of economic savings (Victora et al, 2016).

The federal and state governments within Australia recognise the importance of breastfeeding. The Australian National Breastfeeding Strategy states, 'Nutrition in the first 1000 days is one of the most significant factors that influences child health and development. The nutritional status of the mother and/or child is a critical factor in "programming" the child for healthy development and positive long-term health and wellbeing outcomes' (COAG Health Council, 2019).

An act of love

Breastfeeding is the gift of human kindness. More than a source of nutrition, breastfeeding is an act of altruism, which promotes instincts within the mother to protect and nurture her infant in both the short and long term. Oxytocin is the 'hormone of love' and synthesised in the human brain. Both women and men release oxytocin during lovemaking.

Oxytocin, when released from the posterior pituitary gland, creates a symbiotic effect on the infant and mother, stimulating the 'milk ejection let-down reflex' to feed the baby while causing the uterus to contract, which protects the mother from haemorrhage and aids the involution of the uterus to pre-pregnant size. Hormones released when the mother is stressed or afraid can inhibit the release of oxytocin.

A systematic review of the scientific literature in 2019 included 17 studies, which used mother-infant and/or father-infant play and skin-to-skin contact between maternal-infant and paternal-infant dyads to examine oxytocin's role in early life bonding and parenting processes (Scatliffe et al, 2019). The review concluded that oxytocin has an important role in parental attachment with their infant and promotes bonding and protective instincts between the mother, partner and child. Parents with higher oxytocin levels were shown to exhibit more synchrony and responsiveness in their infant interactions.

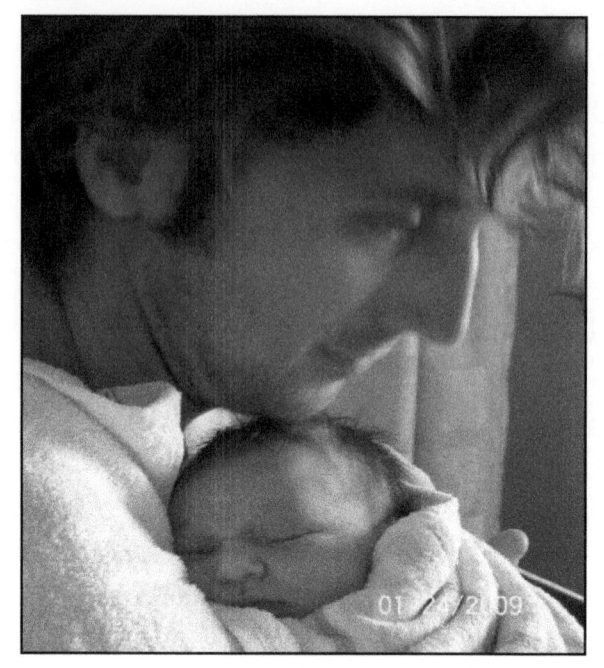

New born and father following birth

Trust and attachment

In a large research study in Queensland, Doctor Lane Strathearn demonstrated that breastfeeding provides a fourfold protection against maternal neglect (Strathearn et al, 2009). When an infant is born, the quality of care given by the caregiver is responsible for wiring the rapidly growing infant's brain. As consistent care builds trust and protects the infant, a secure attachment is important so that, when in danger, the infant knows who to seek for protection. When Doctor King and others introduced infant-feeding schedules, they effectively shut down the evolutionary protective biological hormones needed to promote breastmilk production and the protective bonding and mothering instincts of secure attachment.

Studies using saliva testing to measure stress hormones in an infant when separated from a caregiver, as well as MRI imaging on both parent and child, have demonstrated that securely attached children have lower cortisol levels and behave differently from insecurely attached children. The evolutionary theory of attachment is one of protection. When the infant is securely attached to a few caregivers, the child will know who they can trust when seeking safety, unlike insecurely attached children, such as those in institutions where caregiving is erratic. Studies have been made of children institutionalised in Romania during the Ceausescu regime in the late twentieth century (Glasper, 2020). How the children developed in subsequent caring situations has been followed ever since. Many of these children had long-term neurological damage due to the amount of time institutionalised and the impact of stress and neglect.

My story: Breastfeeding and male shame

In 2005, I became an international board-certified lactation consultant after practising as a midwife for 25 years. I was amazed by the new knowledge that was available from breastfeeding researchers and educators. Unfortunately, up-to-date scientific breastfeeding information has not been adequately disseminated into the wider community because breastfeeding does not fit the capitalist model. Conservative white males, while happy to support a squad of slightly clad cheerleaders at a football match, will complain when a women wants to breastfeed her baby.

One beautiful spring day I went into the public toilets at the races and spoke with a mother who was breastfeeding in the cold and dark room adjacent to the toilets. When I asked her why she was not feeding her baby in the sunshine she said she thought she would be chastised if she did so. While there are public advertising campaigns on many health issues, such as driving without a seatbelt or under the influence of alcohol, much of the public remain unaware that a woman has the right to feed their infant when hungry.

Researcher Karen Epstein-Gilboa (2006) has reported upon the gender differences of parenting styles and reported that the quality of support that nursing mothers receive affects their capacity and resolve to push through the difficulties sometimes associated with breastfeeding. When a partner is envious and feels displaced by the infant, support for the mother and infant may be withheld. In resolving envy, it is important that clinicians are educated in the normal physiological and emotional trajectories of becoming a parent.

I have supported many different families in the production of milk and, while most couples are heterosexual, some families are not. One non-birth mother of a gay couple with twins induced lactation after seeing her partner exhausted and struggling. By expressing regularly she built up a supply of 450 millilitres of milk a day. Not only was she able to feed her children but she enhanced her relationship with her partner.

I also cared for a man who had transitioned to female after being referred to me by an endocrinologist. She explained that she was seeking my help to produce breastmilk to show her partner that she was a real woman. The couple had older children from a previous relationship but no baby. I explained to the client that if she wanted to produce more than the 10 millilitres she was currently expressing, she would have to express regularly to increase the supply to make adequate milk for donations to a human milk bank.

The history of infant feeding since women were hospitalised for maternity care reflects the views of physicians of the past and a dominant patriarchal elite, and impacts preventative and environment health. While attending the WHO/UNICEF BFHI country coordinators meetings in Italy and Lithuania in 2010 and 2014, I noted that the chief nutritionist from WHO and the Japanese delegation were the only men in the room. Australia did not have a representative with any significant authority to bring about change.

Allegra Holmes (2017) reported in her thesis that while the female body is designed for the purpose of growing and birthing children, for many the specific politics of motherhood are irrelevant until they become mothers themselves.

****

The extraordinary qualities of breastmilk

Scientists researching breastmilk have found that women produce antibodies when sick or unwell, which are passed through breastmilk to protect their infant. In 2017, Tedros Adhanom Ghebreyesus, the Director-General of WHO said, 'Breastfeeding gives babies the best possible start in life ... Breastmilk works like a baby's first vaccine, protecting infants from potentially deadly diseases and giving them all the nourishment they need to survive and thrive' (WHO, 2017).

Anthropologists researching human milk have found that breastmilk composition across the world changes according to climatic conditions (Quinn et al, 2016; Tomori et al, 2017). Babies in hotter countries do not require extra fluid substitutes as mothers produce adequate fluids when breastfeeding to hydrate their infant while in the cold climates mothers produce milk with higher fat concentration to keep their babies warm (Almroth, 1978).

Breastmilk for mammalian infants is species, age and gender specific. Scientists researching other lactating mammals have learned, for example, that tammar wallabies can feed two different-sized joeys milk from adjacent teats or mammary glands that differs in composition (Parrot et al, 2023). The reproductive strategy of the tammar wallaby includes a short gestation (26 days). The embryo, following birth, attaches to the nipple within the mother wallaby's pouch and develops for 300 days. It is reliant on lactation to grow. While the tiny wallaby is maturing, the mother wallaby can simultaneously feed an older joey on a second nipple inside the pouch, with the two infants receiving different milk to suit their age requirements. The smaller infant receives a more diluted milk, low in fat and protein and high in carbohydrates, while the older animal receives concentrated milk, high in protein and fat.

Different animals have evolved different strategies to feed their infants. Cape fur seals lactate for two to three days when onshore and have repeated lactation cycles while coming and going on foraging trips at sea, where they can remain for up to 28 days.

Scientists have discovered that in primates and bovine mother's milk the milk is different in male and female singleton offspring (Grote et al, 2016; van Sadelhoff et al, 2018). Tests on monkeys and human milk have indicated that the make-up of milk can vary greatly, but there is evidence to show that milk is different for male and female infants. While the reasons for this disparity are unclear, one hypothesis is that females are fast-tracked to mature earlier than males, as they have a shorter reproductive life and, therefore, differing nutritional requirements compared to the male infants. Like most foods, the make-up of the milk also has a direct impact on growth, behaviour and temperament.

Breastfeeding and contraception

The Innocenti Declaration documents, easily found on the Internet, describe how breastfeeding can be used as a contraceptive during the first six months following birth.

Some 98 per cent of women are at risk of becoming pregnant when they have a baby six months or older, as it is around this time that babies begin to eat complementary foods, and breastfeeding hormone levels drop due to reduced breastfeeding. Once women have a return of their periods, are supplementing breastfeeding regularly with other foods or allowing long stretches during the day or night to elapse between breastfeeds, ovulation may occur (see Figure 8.1). Given that it is recommended women take a three-year gap between pregnancies to allow a return to optimum health, a complementary family planning method is necessary.

Figure 8.1: The Lactation Amenorrhea Method for Family Planning: Source: Innocenti declaration, 1990

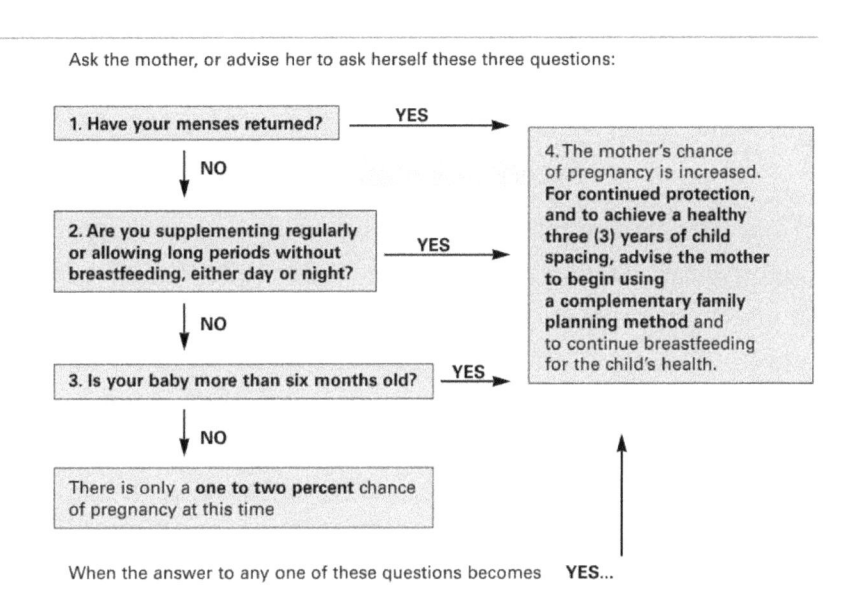

Ask the mother, or advise her to ask herself these three questions:

1. Have your menses returned? — YES →

NO ↓

2. Are you supplementing regularly or allowing long periods without breastfeeding, either day or night? — YES →

NO ↓

3. Is your baby more than six months old? — YES →

NO ↓

There is only a **one to two percent** chance of pregnancy at this time

4. The mother's chance of pregnancy is increased. **For continued protection, and to achieve a healthy three (3) years of child spacing, advise the mother to begin using a complementary family planning method** and to continue breastfeeding for the child's health.

When the answer to any one of these questions becomes YES...

Breastfeeding in emergencies

Breastfeeding is the safest option in emergency situations, and disaster management and strategies need to be put into place to support mothers and infants during these times. Just as staff on an aeroplane or in hospitals are drilled on the appropriate management to save lives, so too must governments be ready with an action plan and not wait until disaster strikes. WHO has written Infant and Young Child Feeding Guidelines for emergency situations but governments around the world are slow to implement them.

Case reports of infant deaths during times of hardship show that mothers become stressed and their supply of breastmilk is reduced. Australia has experienced many emergencies in recent times such as the Black Saturday fires in Victoria in 2009 and the fires that swept through Cobargo during the summer of 2021. Stress is the enemy of breastmilk supply and lactation consultant advice was crucial so that women had the correct strategies to maintain their milk. This is particularly pertinent when alternative milk to feed their infant may not be available.

The logical choice

When infants are weaned they are vulnerable as they no longer have the protective properties provided by breastmilk. When I explained to a teenage couple with a very premature baby in the neo-natal nursery why they should continue giving the mother's own milk and not wean, they became extremely excited. I told them about the unique qualities of breastmilk, and that breastmilk was alive and protected the little one's gut from infection with antibodies. They had been flown in from a rural area with little knowledge and responded to this information saying, 'Wow', and that breastmilk was 'cool'. After discovering the advantages of breastmilk they decided not to wean.

Like many people, they were under the impression that commercial milk and breastmilk were the same.

Spending resources on commercial infant food which may put the lives of infants at risk and undermine a mother's own milk is not a logical choice. However within the health sector four times in my recent memory I have been told in one on one conversations with very influential male doctors, and they would deny what they told me if questioned, that:

1. They would prefer to spend their research time and money on developing a breast milk substitute equivalent to human milk than support breastfeeding women.

2. That if it was their own baby they would prefer to feed commercial infant milk.
3. That I should concentrate on caring for women above the umbilicus and they would care for women below. Which I understood as we will not help support breastfeeding women.
4. That BFHI was not of interest to them and they would leave it to the midwives and lactation consultants. We both knew if he was involved in allocating resources he would not support resourcing breastfeeding women.

And when attending a lecture on infant feeding I was verbally abused during the question time for supporting the case for donor milk human milk and told to give it a rest.

So what is about breastfeeding which causes such division? All of these people know the science and breastmilk is the healthiest option for vulnerable infants but choose to preserve the status quo. Is it a deep seated misogyny, or an aversion to the leaking bodily fluid, or is it envy or greed? Whatever it is, it is not logical.

9

The Economics of Breastfeeding

'Not breastfeeding is associated with lower intelligence and economic losses of about $302 billion annually or 0·49 per cent of world gross national income' (Rollins et al, 2016). James Akre, an author and nutritionist when giving 'one man's perspective' on why he supports breastfeeding, asks his readers to consider that breastmilk has evolved over 260 million years to meet the unique needs of humans (Akre, 2016). Breastmilk makes humans smarter, healthier and more connected, as well as reducing the carbon footprint on the planet.

Economists and environmentalists have shown that breastfeeding is environmentally friendly. Breastfeeding reduces the impact of the dairy industry on the environment by lowering levels of methane and the significant use of water required to produce cow's milk-derived baby milk powders (Smith, 2017). Breastfeeding also reduces waste from feminine hygiene products through delayed menses, and packaging from commercial infant milk cans, bottles and teats. In times of food shortages and national emergencies breastfeeding contributes to food security and is protective of mothers and infants (Tomori, 2023).

In April 2024, the Crawford School's Tax and Transfer Policy Institute at the Australian National University presented a seminar entitled 'Gender responsive budgeting and the financing of maternity care in the Australian Federation: addressing gender equality including in emergencies and disasters'. When following how money was distributed to maternity services in Australia, Charles Maskell-Knight – a retired senior servant with 25 years' experience working in the Department of Health and Ageing – said that a bargain was struck between the Federal Government and states after the Commonwealth promised to provide free health care to Australians. The states owned the 700 public hospitals so the Commonwealth agreed to pay half the monies required to run them. The states agreed because they could not afford not to.

The costs of running the hospitals takes up to a fifth to sixth of a state's budget. The Commonwealth pays a little under half in block grants, which have been adjusted over time to allow for population growth and price changes and are paid weekly into state treasury bank accounts. It is up to the states to determine how much each hospital receives. Each local hospital's network uses activity-based, case-mix accounting systems to forecast the projected levels of activity and monies required. Although there is a projected level of activity determined by maternity units, there is no requirement that the states allocate these monies to the maternity service. Maskell-Knight said greater transparency is required to ensure that best practice is delivered, as activity-based funding provides what is, and not what should be.

Case-mix funding

The Australian Refined Diagnosis Related Groups (AR-DRG) public hospital payment for a woman's care following an uncomplicated caesarean section in 2016 was $9853, compared to $4515 for an uncomplicated normal vaginal delivery. An AR-DRG is a classification system (case-mix) that provides a clinically meaningful way of relating the number and type of patients treated in a hospital to the resources required by the hospital when providing the treatment or care (see Figure 9.1).

Activity-based funding like the current AR-DRG accounting system is not ideal. Better or more cost-effective forms of care may be ignored because big ticket items such as a caesarean section will bring in more money to the institution and doctors in the short term.

While safe caesarean section has saved the lives of countless mothers and babies, a financial incentive to choose caesarean section over vaginal birth may influence the doctor's decision. When separating mothers and babies in the neonatal nursery for around 48 hours. The AR-DRG payment was calculated at $4016 (Scarf V et al, 2021, 2021). Neither performing an unnecessary caesarean section nor separating mothers from their infants is optimum in the short or long term. It is ultimately the woman who pays. In the short term she has to care for her infant with a surgical wound or be separated from her baby, which can increase anxiety levels and impacts on bonding and breastfeeding, her recovery and the ability to care for her baby. She will be dealing with post-operative pain and a longer healing period. The woman is more likely to have a repeat caesarean section in a subsequent pregnancy with risks caused by the uterine scar. The uterine scar may weaken the uterine wall, which can lead to the uterus rupturing, or the placenta may adhere to the uterine wall (placenta accreta). Some women may choose not to have another child because they do not want another caesarean section.

Figure 9.1: Australian Refined Diagnosis Related public hospital costs, 2016–2017. Source: Scarf, 2021

Table 1 AR-DRG definitions included in cost estimations

AR-DRG code[a]	Definition	Cost[b]
O60C	Vaginal delivery (minimal complications, singleton) - including women who had no intervention, or received any of the following: induction or augmentation of labour, epidural analgesia, narcotic pain relief, and/or minor perineal trauma.	$4515
O60B	Vaginal delivery (intermittent complications) - including women who had any of the following: multiple birth, instrumental vaginal birth with vacuum or forceps (not in operating theatre), post-partum haemorrhage (PPH), third or fourth degree perineal tear, episiotomy, or other 'non-severe' complications.	$6108
O01C	Uncomplicated Caesarean section, with or without labour.	$9853
P68D	Admission of neonate >= 37 weeks gestation, with minimal complications requiring observation for around 48 hours	$4016
P68C	Admission of neonate >= 37 weeks gestation, with intermediate complications requiring observation for 2-3 days	$5562

[a]Australian Refined Diagnosis Related Groups Version 5.2 Definitions Manual
[b]IHPA National Hospital Cost Data Collection Australian Public Hospitals 2016-17

It has been almost a century since the ideologies of scientific mothering took hold. Science now demonstrates the importance of human breastmilk for human babies and recognises the long-term economic benefits of breastfeeding. As breastmilk has not been valued as part of the economic equation, has supporting women to breastfeed been estimated in AR-DRG funding? In Australia, in light of the lack of breastfeeding knowledge amongst policy makers and health professionals, manufacturers of commercial baby milk may have an edge as the short-term difference in cost may be a reason why breastfeeding women are not adequately supported. Without transparency to ensure that AR-DRG funding accurately reflects the cost of policies to be implemented at the coal face, and includes the cost benefits of providing evidence-based birthing programs for mothers and breastfeeding for infants, the payments will be wrong because they do not reflect the economic benefits of best practice in the longer term. It takes time for nursing staff to assist women to breastfeed. If the mother cannot care for her baby due to a caesarean section or other complication, how is the baby to be fed? Bottle feeding is an easier and cheaper alternative for time-poor nursing staff and tired mothers; however, it may cause long-term health problems and have environmental implications.

The cost of supporting women to breastfeed on the postnatal ward following different types of birth should be assessed. Currently, on NSW postnatal wards, the care of infants is not counted in patient allocation, and infant and staff ratios. On the postnatal ward, due to the ever-increasing complexity of newly birthed women as a result of higher Caesarean section rates and rapid discharge of normal births, 'Birthrate Plus' scores often demonstrate workload levels higher than the score charts allow, but they continue to be used. 'Birthrate Plus' is a tool used for calculating the required midwifery workforce in NSW. The methodology provides a framework to assess the midwifery hours of care required at a service based on a minimum standard of one-to-one midwifery care for labour and birth. If AR-DRG funding does not account for the cost of the care of a mother who has had a caesarean section, as well as the monitoring and breastfeeding support or care of the baby, it is no surprise that women are dissatisfied with their hospital stay.

My story: An American birthing experience

When my daughter was in the USA, a medicalised hospital model was the only birthing choice offered when she was having her second child. Her first child had been delivered naturally in a birth centre in Sydney. In the USA, her husband's employer's health insurers did not offer a midwifery-led model of care. When the pregnancy was at term, the obstetrician tried to force my daughter, a medically trained doctor who understood the risks of having a post-term infant, into an induction of labour. She had no risk factors that may have endangered the baby, so the doctor and my daughter reached a compromise and agreed she could have daily foetal monitoring checks until the baby arrived. I accompanied her to the obstetrician's rooms to care for her toddler during the appointments and was shocked to see promotion of commercial baby milk gift packs in the waiting room.

Eventually my daughter went into spontaneous labour. Despite being fully dilated and wanting to push when she arrived in the hospital delivery suite, she was forced to endure several attempts to insert an intravenous cannula before hospital staff enabled her to push her baby out. She was a healthy young women having her second baby and there was no clinical indication that a cannula was necessary. She remained in hospital a total of five hours and the hospital bill was US$6500, which she challenged. She was required to pay a nursery fee component, even though she did not use it as the infant never left her side. The hospital accountant explained the charges by saying the nursery needed to remain open just in case it was needed, and asked my daughter why she was challenging the bill when her husband's employer would pay. She replied that it was ultimately the taxpayer who paid. Despite the beautiful aesthetics of the hospital, she was dissatisfied with her American birthing experience. She refused the breakfast that was served on a silver tray by a man in a tuxedo, because she had 'afterbirth pains' and had been ignored on several occasions when asking for pain relief. She said the hospital was money driven and the priorities of care were skewed. Soon after we arrived at the hospital to see the baby, she asked us to take her home via the chemist.

In 2021, the USA had an estimated population of 327 million individuals. Most of those individuals had private health insurance or were covered under a federal program (such as Medicare or Medicaid). About 8.6 per cent of the population were uninsured. Individuals (including those who were uninsured), health insurers, and federal and state governments spent 17.4 per cent of the nation's GDP or around US$4 trillion on various types of health consumption expenditures (HCE) in 2021. Despite this massive cost, maternal and infant mortality and morbidity figures were no better than other developed nations such as Sweden and Japan.

****

Susanna I. Scurry

The challenge for women

New Zealand economist and feminist Marilyn Waring challenged the pathologically selfish and rational 'economic man' when launching 'Counting for Nothing' in the 1980s. Waring worked on a committee for the advancement of women at the United Nations when representing New Zealand as a Member of Parliament. I was at a book launch when Waring said that, while working on the committee, projects that would improve the lives of women were impeded by patriarchal male states, including countries from the Middle East and the Papal State, which argued that by improving the lives of women the family would be destroyed.

But how do you define a family? Families can be very different and can vary in make-up depending on time, place, culture and religion. In the Philippines it was a large mental adjustment to accept that women in one of the homes I was invited to visit were completely under the control of the males of the house and not permitted to go out without being accompanied by a male family member.

Since the 1950s families have evolved. Many young people moved to the cities for education and employment as they lacked opportunities in the rural areas. Australian universities with their large international student population have brought young couples together far from home, creating a global village. To own a home in a large major city requires wealth beyond the reach of many, and young families are often trying to manage in small apartments. They may not know their neighbours and have moved away from family support structures. Economic pressures have required a second income and the return of women to the workplace. Without the contribution and support of family, many mothers are isolated. The high physical and emotional toll paid by women when having children in Australia has reduced the fertility rate and Australia depends on immigration to maintain economic growth.

My story: Growing up in the 1950s

When I was growing up my family consisted of Mum and Dad, a heterosexual couple of mainly English heritage; two brothers; numerous aunts, uncles, cousins; and two elderly grandparents. We owned our own home and lived in a country town, on a big block of land in a house that accommodated my parents, brothers and me, and at different times my grandparents. The town was small with a population of around 400 on the Victorian side of the Murray River. We knew everyone and had close and caring relationships, living within a pushbike ride from relatives and friends. As children, we were given great freedom and watched over by other town parents who kept us safe. The parents would signal between themselves when mischief or danger was looming. Caring for the young and old was done mainly by the women within families as many had given up their wartime employment and returned to the home. In my memory, drunkenness was rife as many of the men had returned from the Second World War damaged and perhaps with survivor guilt. Although the men had returned and held down paid employment it was the women who kept it all together.

****

Gross domestic product

Gross domestic product (GDP) is an accounting method developed to measure domestic production throughout the world. Unfortunately, it does not differentiate between activities that increase a nation's wealth in a sustainable manner, and those that use up and destroy finite resources. The GDP is a clumsy tool and raises the question: who or what is the GDP designed to serve?

The GDP does not value the wealth of goods produced by forests or rivers until they are sold off as timber, irrigation or bottled water, and the countryside is degraded. In destroying the forests and rivers, it is not only the flora and fauna that is devastated, but the quality of life for all of humanity. Meanwhile, the sale of armaments when fighting a war, and insurance payouts when there are bushfires, floods, oil spills or earthquakes, are all calculated in the GDP.

The GDP recognises the paid aged care sector, which contributes one per cent annually to GDP, but does not include the unpaid caring work of parents or family members. The work my mothers and aunts performed at home when caring for children and aged parents was the preferred option for both but not valued by the economic system. This attitude has meant that altruistic care has been pushed to the margins with catastrophic consequences.

My story: Dying at home

My mother refused to go to hospital when she was dying from pancreatic cancer saying she had had enough and they would only hurt her there. Our general practitioner organised a palliative care nurse to keep her pain free with a morphine infusion and my brother and I cared for her at home. She was comforted by the peace and quiet of her own surroundings, and food she preferred to eat. I would sponge her in bed, massaging her feet which she loved. I could brush her hair and we played gentle music. She was not in pain or frightened, and because my brother and I were nearby she could overhear our conversations when resting. We held her hands when she took her last breath while my brother and I supported each other. The way my mother died has been a source of comfort to those left behind. Humans are not individual units; they operate in an interdependent community.

****

Care in the aged and disability sector has shifted from the home to government or private agencies. The high cost of this shift is paid by taxpayers or family members for what, in many cases, is a poor and lesser caring system. The aged care sector has been spotlighted in a Government Inquiry and through the COVID pandemic, and my personal experience is that things have not improved. A family member who had received her letter from the King as she had passed her hundredth birthday lived at home alone, supported by family members who cared for her daily. When she went into a local nursing home because of worsening dementia, she died within three months from bed sores and scabies. These are both preventable and occur as a result of poor nursing and lack of cleanliness. She told her grandson when he visited that she was lonely and left sitting in a chair most of the time, and no longer wanted to live. Another elderly family member in her nineties who had been cared for by her two daughters went into a nursing home where she also died within three months from COVID, which she contracted within the facility.

Because the GDP does not include the unpaid work done by women or another family member when they care, government accounting fails to support altruistic caring. What may be optimum for the individual is invisible in the GDP. Although current estimates value the production of breastmilk within Australia at around AU$3 billion annually, breastfeeding is not supported and women receive few benefits.

Susanna I. Scurry

Ongoing female exploitation

Patriarchy and the capitalist economic model has wedged women who continue to be exploited. They do more than their share of home duties and are, on average, paid less than men when entering the workforce. Because caring work is predominantly performed by women, it is paid at a lesser rate compared to jobs performed by men. These exploitative practices have seen an exodus from caring roles such as teaching, nursing and childcare, and a return to rural areas by young families as property prices are more affordable and give families a more balanced lifestyle. Technological advancements that allow working from home have reduced the reliance on centralisation and, as a result, many Australian cities have lost their heart. Cities without young families and artisans lose their sense of community and vitality.

Cities have become places where only the wealthy can afford to live. The emphasis by government and institutions on money has led to accommodation being sold off and inappropriate development. Nurses and teachers were once supplied subsidised housing close to their workplace by their employers. These essential services providers can no longer afford to live in cities within close proximity to their work, and many have to travel long distances home. One of my colleagues died running off the road after a night shift. Falling asleep is a huge risk when driving home tired and I would often wind down the window or jump out of the car to wake myself up after working through the night.

Robert Kennedy spoke of the failures of GDP when running for president in the USA in 1968, and what he said then holds true today.

> If we believe that we, as Americans, are bound together by a common concern for each other, then an urgent national priority is upon us. We must begin to end the disgrace of this other America ... Our Gross

National Product, now, is over $800 billion dollars a year, but that Gross National Product — if we judge the United States of America by that — that Gross National Product counts air pollution and cigarette advertising, and ambulances to clear our highways of carnage. It counts special locks for our doors and the jails for the people who break them. It counts the destruction of the redwood and the loss of our natural wonder in chaotic sprawl. It counts napalm and counts nuclear warheads and armoured cars for the police to fight the riots in our cities. It counts Whitman's rifle and Speck's knife, and the television programs which glorify violence in order to sell toys to our children. Yet the gross national product does not allow for the health of our children, the quality of their education or the joy of their play. It does not include the beauty of our poetry or the strength of our marriages, the intelligence of our public debate or the integrity of our public officials. It measures neither our wit nor our courage, neither our wisdom nor our learning, neither our compassion nor our devotion to our country, it measures everything in short, except that which makes life worthwhile (Kennedy, 1968).

My story: Institutional care

I remember my mother being outraged when she received a small government payment while caring for her own mother who had dementia and was living at home. She found the payment insulting and said that it barely covered the cost of the cleaning agents she needed when washing the sheets.

At the end of paid parental leave, when women are removed from family, finding and settling a child into a new childcare arrangement can be a difficult adjustment period. When my daughter returned to work, I inspected various childcare centres for the days when I could not care for my granddaughter. I lived several hours travel time from Sydney and could only spare one or two days a week due to other family and work obligations. I was very disappointed by what was on offer in the community. Many of the childcare facilities reminded me of the old people's homes I had worked in as a new nurse, where staffing was in short supply and the smell of human waste permeated the facility. In one place I visited, three infants were lying on a mat on the floor bottle feeding themselves. I came away very depressed. There was no comparison with the one-on-one care I could provide at home.

I recall sitting for several hours with a crying toddler trying to comfort him when working in a paediatric ward on night duty. He was frightened following an operation and wanted his mother. I remember sitting with my own child when he was admitted to hospital and remained because he became stressed when a family member was not present and his condition worsened. I also remember my heartache when separated from my parents when in hospital as a young child.

In PNG, where I worked at the Kimbe hospital, mothers were often seen nursing and cuddling sick children. There it was normal for a family member to remain to provide emotional and physical support for most patients.

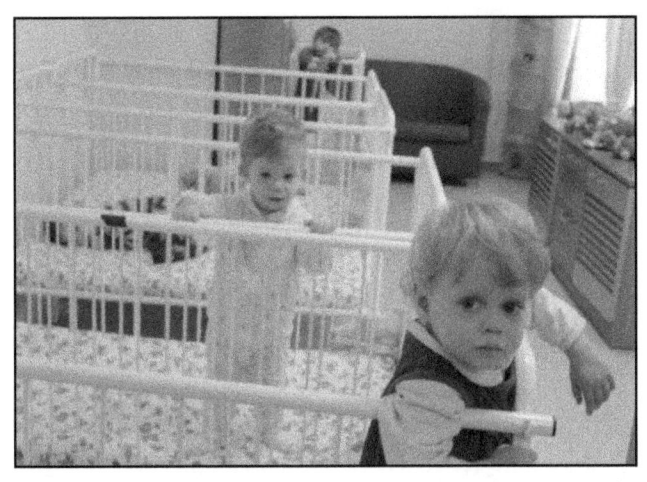

Infants in institutionalised care. What is striking about this photo is that all the infants are alone without physical or emotional stimulation and look lost.

When undertaking research in Japan for this book, I visited a large, privately run maternity hospital with a well-baby nursery on the postnatal ward where healthy newborns were cared for while the mothers recovered following birth. The hospital had a high epidural and caesarean section rate and was run on a medical model with every technological advancement available. However, I could feel my stress levels going up just by being there. While I was on the tour, I looked through the nursery window and watched wakeful babies giving off feeding cues. They were alone and looking around searchingly, with some crying without receiving attention. I also saw mothers alone, wandering the corridors or in private rooms. It is a normal human response for parents to respond to their infants' cues for attention, and separating parents from their infants can mean that both parents and infants can become stressed due to the release of stress hormones. Nils Bergman believes that the mother and infant should not be separated, and the ongoing emotional connection created by skin-to-skin contact is a cornerstone to development and resilience (Bergman, 2019).

****

Finding the right care

I have a friend who cared for her grandchild following her daughter's caesarean section and admission from the operating theatre to intensive care. Her daughter was placed on a respirator because of permanent lung damage from a very premature birth. My friend sat in the hospital nursery cuddling her grandchild and then would sit with her daughter in the intensive care unit. Her daughter was extremely restless and fighting the medications given to sedate her while on the respirator. My friend challenged the hospital rules by asking that she bring the baby to intensive care because she believed the mother would settle if her baby was near. Once the mother and baby were reunited and the baby placed near the mother she relaxed and was soon on the road to recovery.

I have many friends who have sold their family homes in the cities to move to regional areas to be with their children who had already moved as they could no longer afford city prices. My friends care for their grandchildren with mixed emotions. Many have other skills and would be financially better off if they remained in the workforce but believe it is better to be caring for their grandchildren than have them cared for by a stranger. Vasti Calitz, in a Master's thesis entitled, *The exploitation of the labour of love*, concluded that nurturing work allowed an individual to flourish and contributed to the quality of relationships. Many grandparents know this and accept the financial disadvantages because they want to help their children and grandchildren. However, because they are older and the work is tiring, they can feel obligated or resentful.

The cost of breastfeeding

The failure to include the cost of the time women invest producing breastmilk when calculating the GDP has led to a lack of support for mothers and infants in the capitalist model. The cost of breastmilk can be valued. A healthy baby will drink 30 millilitres of milk per kilo of their weight every three to four hours. Pasteurised donor milk was on sale recently in Australia at AUD15 per 100 millilitres. A 3-kilogram baby will drink around 100 millilitres every three to four hours. Using the cost from the donor milk sale, the value of breastmilk is AU$120 in a 24-hour period. If the mother feeds to WHO recommendations, an infant will be exclusively breastfed for around six months, which makes a mother's contribution to the economy AUD$21,840. As the infant gains weight and consumes more milk, the cost of milk increases.

Compare the cost of commercial baby milk at supermarket prices. A can of baby milk powder is on average AU$22. If a baby weighs 3 kilograms and drinks around 100 millilitres every three to four hours, a can of powdered baby milk will last for around a week. The total value of commercial milk powder is significantly less than breastmilk and is around AU$572 for six months.

The AR-DRG classification system pays the greatest amount for the care of mothers and babies within the highest intervention category, which may mean women are pushed into care they would prefer not to have. It is easy to manipulate women when they think their infant may be at risk. In Japan, the prefectures pay women a maternity stipend when the pregnancy is at around 18 weeks gestation, which gives women the opportunity to choose the maternity care that best suits them. In Australia, women have little autonomy over their birth decisions.

Failure of the GDP

Nobel Prize-winning economists Amartya Sen and Joseph Stiglitz have pointed out the flawed nature of the GDP. The emphasis on wealth creation has created exploitative practices in a bid for larger profits. Women have been discriminated against and are fed up with the unequal treatment they receive. Within Australia, women with education and choice have sought changes that lighten their load. These changes may include choosing a partner who recognises women as equals or choosing sperm from a catalogue and having a child alone or moving into the paid workforce and reducing their caring load. The GDP and the current capitalist model demands too much in its avarice and has impinged on altruism to a point where most carers have stopped caring. It is clearly an outdated tool.

A society that does not value the freely given altruistic work undertaken by a mother or father to raise a secure child, or the unpaid kindnesses of grandparents to care for their grandchildren, or the freely given work done by a family member in caring for the sick, disabled or elderly relative or friend at home is a sad society. I cannot overemphasise how important the support of the grandparents, aunts, uncles and other mothers were to me as a new mother with five children under the age of nine. They all contributed to turning out five great assets, who have gone on to have children of their own while giving back to society.

10

Improving Breastfeeding Rates

In 2007, breastfeeding advocates were full of hope. The Australian parliamentary inquiry into breastfeeding had listened to breastfeeding women and other relevant parties throughout the country. In 2008, 22 recommendations were made. Only Recommendations 5 and 10 were implemented:

> Recommendation 5: That the Department of Health and Ageing fund the Australian Breastfeeding Association to expand its current breastfeeding helpline to become a toll-free national breastfeeding helpline
>
> Recommendation 10: That the Speaker of the House of Representatives and the President of the Senate take the appropriate measures to enable the formal accreditation by the Australian Breastfeeding Association of Parliament House as a Breastfeeding Friendly Workplace (Commonwealth of Australia, 2007).

Falling breastfeeding rates

Breastfeeding is not rocket science and significant gains could be made with a genuine, systematic approach. The Australian National Breastfeeding Strategy: 2019 and Beyond presents a pathway to achieving the SDG targets.

Women want to breastfeed and breastfeeding initiation rates in Australia are high. When women birthed at home under the care of independent midwives and other women, breastfeeding was the norm. When birthing and breastfeeding became scientific and women were hospitalised, breastfeeding rates declined. In a baseline survey of breastfeeding rates undertaken by the Australian Institute of Health and Welfare in 2010, 96 per cent of women were shown to have initiated breastfeeding. At one month, the same survey found that exclusive breastfeeding rates had fallen to 61.4 per cent of babies, and by five to six months of the infant's age, 15 per cent of infants were exclusively breastfeeding. These figures are well short of the SDG targets for 2030, which aims for 50 per cent of infants being exclusively breastfed at around six months of age and demonstrate the system is broken.

Breastfeeding rates fall in differing amounts when women undertake part or full-time work. The lack of support for breastfeeding in the workplace is a barrier for women. A breastfeeding childcare worker I know was so needed by her employers because of staff shortages following the COVID pandemic, they made a place available for her baby within the childcare centre where she worked to induce her to return to work early. This scenario demonstrates that by creating an enabling environment within the workplace women can continue to work and breastfeed.

Figure 10.1 is a comparison of exclusive breastfeeding and mixed feeding from birth until six months of the infant's age, based on research conducted in Australia following a parliamentary inquiry into breastfeeding in 2010.

Figure 10.1: Proportion of children exclusively breastfed (bottom line) and a proportion of children partially breastfeeding (top line) at each month of age in 2010 (percentage). Source: Australian Institute of Health and Welfare

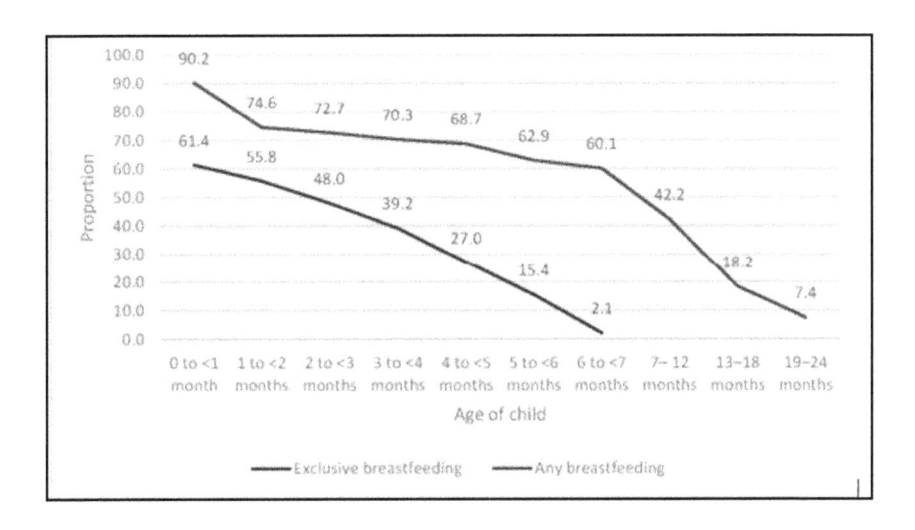

A change in rates

A national health survey conducted by the Australian Bureau of Statistics from August 2020 to June 2021 during the COVID pandemic demonstrates that breastfeeding rates had improved since the 2010 report (see Figure 10.2). The survey collected data from 1100 households and focused on the health status of Australians and health-related aspects of lifestyles of Australian families. Due to the Covid pandemic, data was collected via a self-completed online form with no face-to-face interviews, and may have excluded some non-English-speaking households. The 2020–2021 survey demonstrated higher breastfeeding rates occur when women are given time and access to their infants. This survey provides anecdotal evidence that women who have more time at home (in this case, due to the mandatory lockdowns) will breastfeed if given the opportunity.

Figure 10.2: Proportion of children aged 0–3 years who were exclusively breastfed for 2, 4 and 6 months, 2020–2021. Source: Australian Institute of Health and Welfare

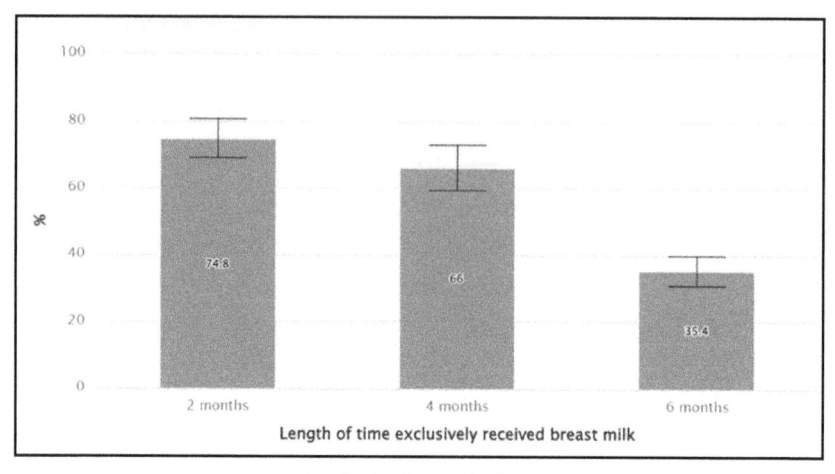

Exclusive breastfeeding

Paid maternity leave

In 2009, I appeared as a witness before the Productivity Commission to help argue the case for women to receive six months paid maternity leave. Evidence demonstrated that many women returning to work and leaving their baby for paid employment became anxious and depressed. In the past, a family could afford to live comfortably on one income and women could remain at home to breastfeed. Before the productivity commission inquiry, as a member of the Australian Lactation Consultants Association, I made representation to the Australian Council of Trade Unions, with evidence from WHO and recommendations for optimum infant outcomes when breastfeeding. Many witnesses appeared before the commission to give evidence, including Decalie Brown, President of the International Lactation Consultants Association. Prior to the hearing, commentators were predicting the outcome would be three months paid maternity leave but, to the surprise of many, the Commission recommended four months.

With the election of the Albanese-led Labor Government in 2022, paid maternity leave increased to six months. This is in line with the Global Strategy for Infant and Young Child Feeding, which has four operational targets (Innocenti Declaration, 1990).

1. Appoint a national breastfeeding coordinator with appropriate authority and establish a multisector national breastfeeding committee composed of representatives from relevant government departments, non-governmental organisations, and health professional associations.
2. Ensure that every facility providing maternity services fully practises all the Ten Steps to Successful Breastfeeding set out in the WHO/UNICEF statement on breastfeeding and maternity services.
3. Give effect to the principles and aim of the International Code of Marketing of Breast-Milk Substitutes and subsequent relevant Health Assembly resolutions in their entirety.
4. Enact imaginative legislation protecting the breastfeeding rights of working women and establish means for its enforcement.

The Declaration states that babies should be exclusively breastfed until around six months of age, when appropriate complementary foods can be introduced with continued breastfeeding for two years or more. From July 2023, paid parental leave in Australia transitioned from 18 weeks to 20 weeks, with subsequent two-weekly increases to be paid each year, until a total of 26 weeks of paid parental leave is reached. The current change to implement six months paid maternity leave is a positive step for young families and welcomed by breastfeeding advocates. Giving mothers financial support during the first year following the birth of a baby is an act of compassion and respect for the valuable contribution made by women to the nation.

Figure 10.3: Breastfeeding practices and determinants. Source: Hector, 2005

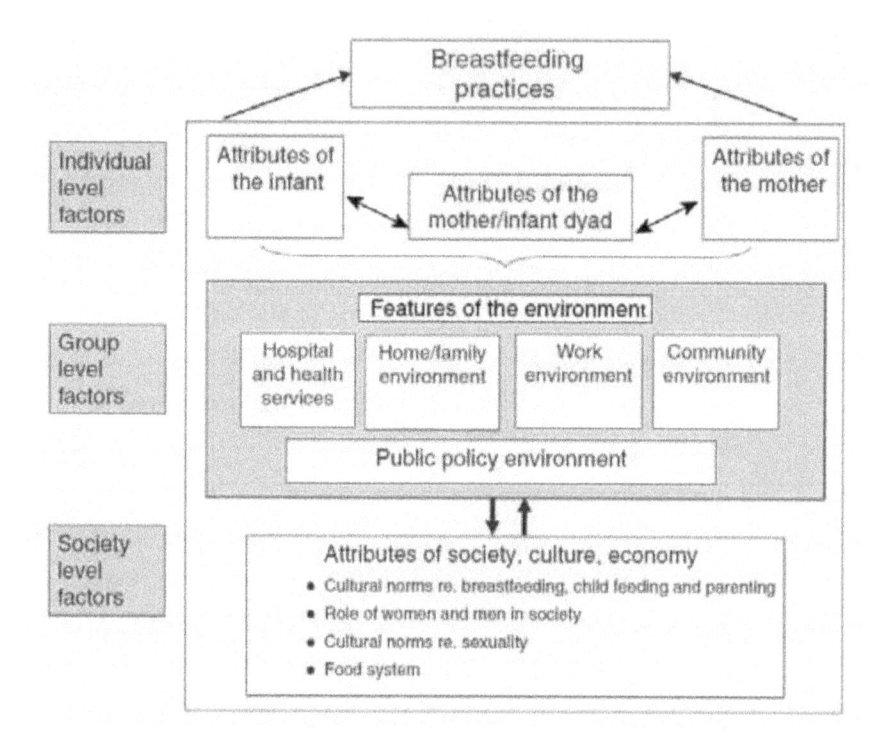

```
                          ┌──────────────────┐
                          │  Breastfeeding   │
                          │    practices     │
                          └──────────────────┘
┌──────────┐  ┌──────────────┐                    ┌──────────────┐
│Individual│  │ Attributes of│                    │ Attributes of│
│  level   │  │  the infant  │──Attributes of the─│  the mother  │
│ factors  │  │              │  mother/infant dyad│              │
└──────────┘  └──────────────┘                    └──────────────┘

              ┌────────────────────────────────────────────────┐
              │         Features of the environment            │
┌──────────┐  │ ┌────────┐ ┌──────────┐ ┌────────┐ ┌─────────┐ │
│  Group   │  │ │Hospital│ │Home/     │ │ Work   │ │Community│ │
│  level   │  │ │and     │ │family    │ │environ-│ │environ- │ │
│ factors  │  │ │health  │ │environ-  │ │ment    │ │ment     │ │
└──────────┘  │ │services│ │ment      │ │        │ │         │ │
              │ └────────┘ └──────────┘ └────────┘ └─────────┘ │
              │         Public policy environment              │
              └────────────────────────────────────────────────┘

┌──────────┐  ┌────────────────────────────────────────────────┐
│ Society  │  │    Attributes of society, culture, economy     │
│  level   │  │  • Cultural norms re. breastfeeding, child     │
│ factors  │  │    feeding and parenting                       │
└──────────┘  │  • Role of women and men in society            │
              │  • Cultural norms re. sexuality                │
              │  • Food system                                 │
              └────────────────────────────────────────────────┘
```

The success or failure of breastfeeding should not be seen solely as the responsibility of the mother. Her ability to breastfeed is very much shaped by the support and the environment in which she lives. There is a broader responsibility of governments and society to support women through policies and programmes in the community.

Multifactorial determinants of breastfeeding need supportive measures at many levels, from legal and policy directives to social attitudes and values, women's work and employment conditions, and health-care services to enable women to breastfeed. When relevant interventions are delivered adequately, breastfeeding practices are responsive and can improve rapidly. The best outcomes are achieved when interventions are implemented concurrently through several channels (Rollins, 2016).

Making infant feeding choices

There are many factors that influence a new mother when it comes to infant feeding choices. If she is supported to breastfeed following the birth by professionals, her partner, family, friends, culture and workplace she will, in most cases, achieve her goals. Lack of support is the main reason women give for not breastfeeding.

Distance and COVID lockdowns have meant the support systems of the past have diminished. The family of one of my children's partners lives in Wales, and when her baby was born being separated from her family made it particularly hard. While technology has improved connectivity, it cannot replace the hands-on help or touch of a loved one when tired or in pain.

My story: The importance of support

When planning her hospital discharge home following mastitis and a breast abscess, a young woman told me that prior to her re-admission to hospital she had been so unwell at home that she could not think, and the support of her partner and mother had saved her life. She was re-admitted to a public hospital rather than the private hospital where her baby had been born because she was very sick. However, she and her partner had found the surgical teams care in the public hospital fragmented and uncaring, showing little interest in her as a breastfeeding mother. While the surgical team treated her infection and drained the abscess, both parents said the doctors had little knowledge of lactation and their consultations were hurried, dismissive and rude.

It had been the midwives, lactation consultants and her family who had advocated for her to ensure that she and the baby were provided with the holistic care needed while she was unable to care for herself. She said while the midwives had nursed her and lactation consultants had attended her breast care and breastfeeding issues, her partner had remained in hospital as her advocate while her mother had cared for the baby overnight at home to allow her to rest and heal. Her mother had fed expressed breastmilk to the baby and encouraged her daughter to breastfeed when she brought the baby to the hospital each day.

The new mother spoke of her partner and mother with admiration and awe. She also spoke about what an awful teenager she had been and how she had treated her mother with a lack of respect. She acknowledged her foolishness, saying her mother had a wealth of knowledge, and could have castigated her but never did. The new mother explained that she felt she had passed through a door, which had given her insight into what it is to be a mother. She does not know how women manage alone and believed the importance of having a caring, supportive network could not be over-emphasised.

****

The need for breastfeeding support

The priority populations where support is needed to improve breastfeeding rates are listed in the Australian National Breastfeeding Strategy, and include Indigenous Australians, linguistically and culturally diverse women, migrants, refugees, asylum seekers, young mothers (teenagers from child bearing age until around 25), and women of low socio-economic background or of a lower level of education. Most of these women are inadequately resourced or may have come from a background of hardship and can ill afford to give commercial baby milk to their infants.

Research shows many reasons for women and babies being at risk of not breastfeeding (see Figure 10.4). Women who work either full-time or part-time, teenagers, older mothers, single mothers, smokers, women with a high body mass index, and women who have had a caesarean section or obstetric complications such as a postpartum haemorrhage. Pre-term babies or babies housed within the neonatal unit and separated from their mothers also have poor breastfeeding outcomes. Strategies to increase breastfeeding rates within these vulnerable groups would not only reduce inequity but would provide short- and long-term cost savings.

While a mother may have all the necessary attributes to breastfeed, the baby may not. Prematurity, illness, jaundice or a congenital abnormality such as a cleft palate or cardiac issue may require extra measures to be put into place to support the mother/baby dyad. Specialist breastfeeding help may be required. In BFHI-accredited and neo-BFHI-accredited health facilities, the accreditation process requires adequate education of health professionals, and knowledge and policies to support these challenging lactation situations.

Figure 10.4: Attributes of the mother and baby at risk of not breastfeeding

Mother	Baby
Age, teenage/older mother	Health status, infection or sick baby
Parity	Gestational Age at birth (prematurity)

Health status, diabetes, postpartum haemorrhage, PCOS or other endocrine disorders such as diabetes	Intrauterine growth retarded infants (IUGR)
Type of birth, Caesarean section, forceps	Multiples such as twins, triplets
Obesity	Congenital abnormalities such as cleft lip or palate, chromosomal disorders, for example Trisomy 21
Breast surgery/aplastic breasts	Jaundice/sleepy babies
Smoking status	Infants of mothers in jail or detention
Culture/Indigenous women/ Linguistically diverse	
Marital status	

In my home in Stockton, there is a lot of subsidised government housing, with many poorly educated and lower socio-economic families. My husband related a scenario he had seen occur on the ferry when he was returning from work. A new mother from the social housing was sitting near him with her baby in the pram. She was discussing infant feeding with a friend who had asked, 'Boob or bottle?' He said the baby's mother despairingly answered, 'I shoulda, I shoulda, I shoulda breastfed', while gesticulating wildly with her hands. 'Not only do I have to carry around all this shit' – she pointed to the bottles, teats, can of formula and nappy bag at the bottom of the pram – 'but it costs!' she said.

My story: An American parent-education day centre

When my grandson was born in the USA, I visited a facility in California and was inspired. My daughter and her toddler attended a council-run parent education day facility centre, Parents' Place, set up in local parklands and paid for by residents' rates. My daughter was far from home with a toddler, expecting a second child and new to the area. She attended the facility with her toddler to be with other parents and children. The facility was the brainchild of a lactation consultant and had the support of other professionals, such as social workers, physiotherapists, childcare workers and artisans. While the parents could obtain help from professionals and mix with other parents, the children heard stories from the *Cat in the Hat*, made mudpies, painted, learned to make pancakes and how to squeeze fresh orange juice.

When visiting Parents' Place, I spoke with a father whose wife was at home dying from breast cancer. He told me he had not only brought his child to Parents' Place to get out of the house for a while and socialise with other parents, but also to bring his child to a place of fun and happiness. I also met a mother of 2-year-old twin girls. Her life had been thrown into turmoil since their birth and she told me the facility kept her sane. I was impressed by the helpful information supplied to parents. For example, a poster that said HALT with a crying baby's face was a useful prompt for tired parents. H-hunger, A-attention, L-love and T –tired. I tell new parents about HALT on a daily basis, with strategies to address each letter. When a parent is anxious and tired, a crying child can cause great stress that may result in harm, and these are useful strategies that can help.

****

Transitioning into motherhood

Psychologists recognise differing stages when transitioning to motherhood following birth. Reva Rubin identified three phases she described as 'taking in, taking hold, and letting go' (Rubin, 1967 a and b). Rubin's theory of mothering describes the first three days after giving birth as a time when the mother needs to focus on her own needs of sleep and food while she debriefs to her carers about what has occurred. The next four to 10 days are described by Rubin as a period of taking hold, as the mother becomes more independent after having rested and is ready to assume the tasks of mothering. At this time, she is better able to take in education and learn the skills necessary for mothering. As the average hospital stay in Australia is two to three days, most women will have gone home before being ready to take hold.

In NSW, there is a gap in maternal and infant care that has not been adequately recognised and evaluated. We know that following birth there are high initiation rates of breastfeeding but within the first month exclusive breastfeeding rates fall dramatically. Postnatal care has changed over the decades from a 10-day hospital stay to the present two to three days. The 10-day stay gave women time to transition through the rest and recovery phase and onto the taking hold stage. However, the hospital environment and medical model of care, which excluded partners after visiting hours, and did not keep mothers and infants together so they could learn to breastfeed and care for their infant, failed to address issues that were important to women. Postnatal care has remained on the lowest rung of the childbirth hierarchy for decades. When in the final stages of writing this book my friend Mary told me this story and agreed to write it down for inclusion here.

> My eldest son Nico was born in the afternoon of 15 July 1970. He was small – just over six pounds. My

Patriarchy, Misogyny and Breastfeeding

fault! I was a smoker and did not know it was bad for babies in utero. Nico was smaller than he should have been. We were living in Kensington at the time and my local hospital was Fulham in west London.

After the birth I was taken to a ward of new mothers. There were a dozen of us, I think. My first thought was feeding my first born. I was anxious to start but the nurse on duty told me I had to wait for my milk to come in. I knew nothing about colostrum. In fact, looking back I realise I knew nothing about looking after a newborn baby. I have no idea whether there were classes available at the time for expectant mothers. If there were, I wasn't told by my GP.

At the time, mothers and babies spent a week in hospital. During the day babies were wheeled into the ward in a small cot and left beside their mothers. The nurses handed out small bottles of milk at feeding times. Each time a bottle was placed on the locker beside my bed, I asked when I could start breast feeding. Every time I had the same answer, 'When your milk comes in'. Only one other mother in the ward was as anxious as I was to breastfeed. She was French and found it hard to communicate but her determination to breastfeed was clear. She was given the same brush-off as me.

I think that apart from the staff nurse in charge, all the nurses in that ward were from local agencies. When pressed about breastfeeding they gave the impression that it was simply too much trouble. On the third day after Nico was born, one of the nurses walked round the ward from bed to bed and placed a pill on each locker. When she came to me, I asked what the pill was for. 'It's for drying up your milk', she said. I warned the French mother not to take it. We both threw the pill in our wastepaper bin.

That evening I decided to try my hand at breast feeding on my own. It was hard. I didn't realise I had an inverted nipple which didn't help. There was a different nurse on duty that night and she saw me struggling. She came and sat on my bed and helped me to attach Nico to my bloated boob. It wasn't easy but with persistence, it worked and finally, finally I succeeded. I breastfed Nico for the next six months.

In Australia, following birth, hospital stays have been reduced despite research that demonstrates there is a problem. When my brother was born in the 1960s, my mother remained in hospital for around 10 days. In 1975, when my first child was born, I also remained in hospital for 10 days. In the current situation, a woman may leave hospital within hours of the birth or remain for up to five days following a caesarean section. Many women are forced to leave hospital when they are not ready due to a lack of maternity beds.

I am not advocating a change to longer stays as such; hospitals are not ideal for women. However, hospital stays need to be flexible. When women experience difficulties, it is not easy to access post-hospital discharge live-in support. While women may receive a daily home visit from the hospital maternity service (HMS) for up to five days post birth, midwives are on a time schedule for each visit. Breastfeeding issues take time to resolve and within the public sector midwives have varying experience and skill levels. If an HMS midwife is unsure of when the mother and baby will be seen again, a bottle may be the easiest option to ensure that the infant is getting adequately fed. When I was doing home visiting during a randomised control trial (see Chapter 11), the HMS midwives were very grateful that I had been – or was going to – a woman on their list. A lactation home visit reduced the workload of the HMS midwife.

Australia's fertility rates

Figure 10.5: Total fertility rates 1933–2021. Source: ABS

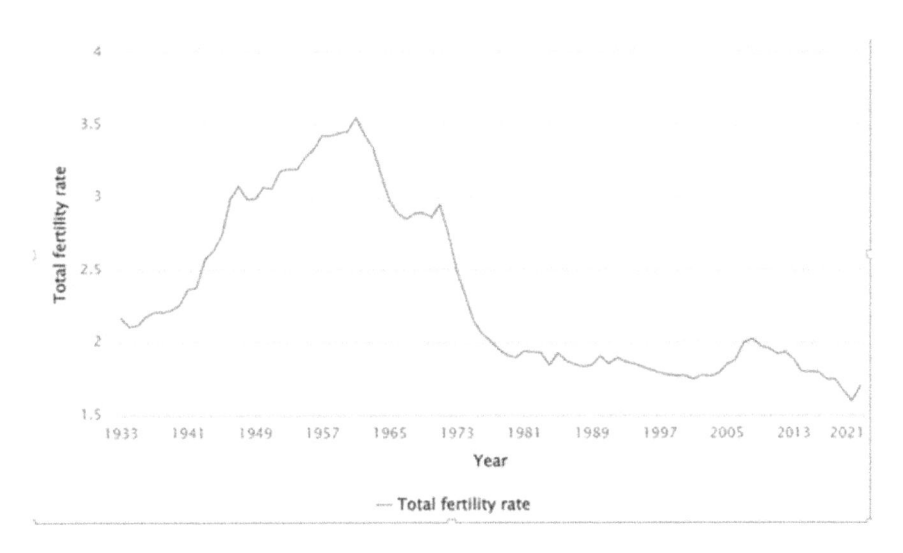

Educated women are choosing to have smaller families and since women were given the freedom to choose the size of their family, birth rates have plummeted (see Figure 10.5). On 7 January 2023, the *Sydney Morning Herald* reported on Australia's low birth rate and quoted first-time mother of eight-month-old Lewis, Ashlee Douglas, as saying all the mothers in her group were debating the size of their families. Ashlee said, 'Plenty of other mothers were tossing up whether to have a second baby. I don't reckon I'll have another, and a lot of mums are saying the same thing' (*Sydney Morning Herald*, 2023).

In 2020, the Australian Bureau of Statistics reported Australia's population base at 1.58 per woman, the lowest rate ever reported and well below the replacement rate of 2.1 (the rate needed for a generation to replace itself). The total fertility rate is a measure that gives the average number of children a woman would have during her lifetime. During the COVID pandemic in 2021, Australia's fertility rate increased marginally to 1.7 while breastfeeding rates increased. These figures demonstrate that with more time and financial pressures removed, in this case due to the COVID lockdowns and subsidised financial arrangements, families will increase in size.

In Australia, rather than implementing measures to support women and implement programs to reduce the caesarean section rate and promote, for example, free childcare, workplace reform, programs to normalise breastfeeding in schools and universities, and lactation home visits until new mothers can drive, Australia will rely on an immigration program to supplement Australia's low fertility rate. In contrast, because Japan's fertility rate is the lowest in the world and the caesarean section rate is 20 per cent, measures to support women are in place in the community. In Israel, the caesarean section rate is 16.1 per cent.

The reason for the disparity in surgical birth numbers throughout the wealthier nations raises a question still to be answered. As the research evidence increases and demonstrates the many disadvantages of an operative delivery for women, the current inquiry in NSW into obstetric violence is of the utmost relevance. In seeking answers, it is important to consider the historical implications of how maternity care in Australia came about.

While many migrant workers are employed in lowly paid jobs and drive economic growth in Australia, they often lack resources or do not speak English, which places them at a disadvantage when institutionalised. I cared for a young migrant woman on the postnatal ward who crawled up into a ball and cried following the birth of her baby. She told me she needed her mother's help following her caesarean section. This is not an uncommon situation.

In NSW, most women receive HMS within the first five days following birth. One home visit by the maternal and child health nurse is scheduled during the first few weeks following birth, and subsequent care is shared between the maternal and child health nurses and general practitioners. Wendy Brodribb, a researcher in Queensland, found general practitioners' knowledge was often dependent upon personal experience and interest (Brodribb et al, 2009). Like general practitioners, child and family health nurses have varying degrees of breastfeeding knowledge. While some child and family health nurses may have had lactation consultant training, others do not.

Parents are issued with a Blue Book in hospital and are expected to have their infants checked at birth, and again by the general practitioner or child and family health nurse at 1 to 4 weeks, 6 to 8 weeks and at 6 to 12 months. For many parents, leaving the house with a baby can be difficult, and for families without a car accessing services may be impossible.

The changes I have seen throughout my lifetime, as a mother and as a health professional, are the result of a top-down approach, mainly from men wanting to control women. The public/private model of maternity care in Australia has been set up often without the input of consumers and to benefit the institution and doctors. In 2021, when undertaking a Master's thesis into the breastfeeding environment of the postnatal ward at the facility where I worked, I researched parent input into the design of a new maternity hospital. Shortly after setting up a breastfeeding clinic, women were asked to share their experiences of the clinic. They described how difficult it was to find a park at the clinic site and how they had weaned because the waiting list to see a lactation consultant was too long. Without consumer input institutions cannot achieve the best outcomes for women.

Governments, through federal- and state-run health departments, and hospitals managed by churches and universities, have created silos that do not practise holistic care. Women have little say in decisions that affect them and their infants, or how their tax health dollar could be better used. They have been dissatisfied for decades with the unequal treatment they receive within the workplace and economic model, and it is not surprising Australian women are choosing to have fewer children. The current price women pay as a result of having children is unfairly distributed within the population. Why should women be forced to live with less money than their male counterparts because their sex determines they have a baby, and when all of society benefits from healthy and well-educated children?

Finland and Japan

The Finnish model of community family care has been highly successful (Grym and Borgermans, 2018a). Maternal and infant mortality and morbidity statistics make Finland the safest place in the world to have a baby. The maternity and child clinics have five primary aims.

1. To promote the health and wellbeing of pregnant people and their families.
2. To reduce health inequalities in society.
3. To monitor and support healthy pregnancy and the growth and development of children.
4. To identify any need for special support as early as possible.
5. To provide support and assistance when needed.

The Finnish model recognises that the transition to motherhood takes time, and women and families are supported throughout their journey. The healthcare model is designed to foster communication between practitioners and families, while building a safe and calm environment to help parents be heard and have agency. In Finland, generous paid maternity and paternity leave reduces the financial pressures on families with a baby.

In 2020, Finland had a maternal death rate of three maternal deaths in 100,000 births. Japan and Sweden each had a rate of four maternal deaths per 100,000 births. The maternal death rate in Australia was 5.5 deaths per 100,000, and in the United States 32.9 deaths per 100,000 births.

Finland recorded 1.42 deaths per 1000 infants, and Japan recorded 1.56 deaths per 1000 infants in 2020. In the same year, infant mortality in Australia and the United States was recorded as higher, on a population basis, than other OECD countries. In Australia, 2.73 deaths occurred per 1000 infants; in the United States 5.48 infant deaths per 1000 births were recorded.

In 2017, Japanese prefectures adopted the Finnish model of care to improve outcomes for families due to high maternal depression, maternal suicide and domestic violence rates (Shimomura, 2017). Japan has an excellent health system, little immigration, the lowest birth rate in the world and an ageing population where people are living into their nineties. Young people have moved to the cities to find work, are living in small apartments and separated from family support structures, all of which have been exacerbated by COVID-19.

In Japan, the prefectures or local councils pay mothers a maternity stipend at around 18 weeks of pregnancy, and the pregnant woman can choose the type of birthing care she wants and best suits her family situation. There is a focus on transitioning to motherhood and families are supported to become families. Following birth, Japanese mothers have seven days of supported postnatal care. They may choose to remain within the midwifery service or hospital, or go home. If the baby is a first child, or the birth has been difficult or an operative birth, or the mother needs time to recover from the epidural anaesthetic (a popular form of pain relief in Japan), the mother may remain where she birthed if she has no help at home, or go home to rest and recover if her partner or family are available to assist with baby care. When the mother is feeling better and ready to take on the care of the baby, or her partner or family can no longer assist, she can elect to be re-admitted to a live-in postnatal facility within her community. There, under the guidance of health professionals, she can learn to care for her baby.

Raising a child is overwhelming and exhausting and requires many hands. When in Japan, I saw examples of how mothers were being supported to raise an only child in community-based facilities amongst other parents. Being the parent of an only child can be not only exhausting but, as shown in the Chinese one-child policy, produce demanding and lonely children in the short term (Cai and Feng, 2021). In both Finland and Japan interventions are provided to support all families, including those at higher risk (for example teenage or single mothers, refugees, chemically dependent women) until children begin school. For some vulnerable women, such as refugees or women from lower socio-economic groups, both the Finnish and Japanese models have introduced programs to help mothers achieve financial independence.

In one of the facilities I visited in Japan, a young mother was employed within the staff, training as a childcare worker. She brought her young son to work where he was cared for in the facility's young child program. The ultimate goal was to have the mother ready to enter the workplace as a trained childcare assistant when the little boy began school. In Japan, I visited several day care centres where women could come and see a health professional, attend a parent group with other parents, have lunch and then leave their infant with nursing staff while going to a quiet area for an afternoon sleep. Mothers were welcome to bring their babies to the community care centres to catch up on sleep until the infant was 4 months of age.

In Finland, *Neuvola* is a program provided from pregnancy through to the start of school that offers optimal care and the time to give women the skills necessary to mother. In learning to love and respect themselves, women grow and develop confidence in their own abilities, which tip over into love for baby and family (Grym and and Borgermans, 2018b).

Australia

Japan and Australia have some similarities, with low birth rates and young families isolated and removed from family support structures having moved to large cities for work and education. Cost of housing in major cities requires some people to live in small apartments, which can be difficult with a crying baby and offer little room for an extra support person. Many young families struggle and the vast distances to be travelled to get help may be impractical. Following the birth of twin nieces, a friend travelled on several occasions from NSW to Western Australia to help her sister-in-law with the premature babies after hospital discharge. Eventually, because of lack of support at home, the mother was admitted to a managed residential care facility, where she received help from healthcare providers while my friend could return home to her own children.

As many of the volunteer support structures that helped mothers in the past no longer exist, the emotional toll placed on parents when leaving their infant in the care of a stranger to enable paid work is too hard. I recall my toddler grandchildren becoming increasing distressed when they recognised their mother was going to work and how they loved remaining at home when a trusted family member was available to stay with them.

In my experience supporting new families, parents may want to have larger families, but the need to put a roof over their heads and afford a decent life and future for their children is limiting. In the past, due to patriarchal ideology, religious pressures or lack of contraception, women had little choice. The development of the contraceptive pill has meant, that since the 1970s, people have had the freedom to choose if and when they want children, as well as family size.

Men in control

The development of agricultural farming led to a desire for men to dominate and form groups to protect land and animals from competitors. Political and religious hierarchies were formed, and women were relegated to subservient positions, with men making decisions and controlling women. Laws were passed that perpetuated the dominance of men and excluded women from positions of power and education, entrenching the claims of male superiority.

If change is to happen, men need to be included in the discussion and given correct and up-to-date knowledge about birthing and breastfeeding. Many men I am in contact with are extremely interested and do want to help their partners when having a new baby. Having a healthy family is important to them. While the intimacies of birth and breastfeeding may be too much information for some, having correct information allows an informed decision that benefits their families.

11

EQUIP: A continuity of care randomised control trial pilot research study

In 2022, I provided lactation support in EQUIP: A continuity of care randomised control trial (RCT) pilot research study conducted by Hunter Medical Research Institute and Newcastle University, which commenced with two groups each of 60 women planning to breastfeed. The aim of the study was to compare the breastfeeding experiences of newly birthed breastfeeding women when provided with a support intervention from birth until the baby was six months of age. Continuity of care with a known international board-certified lactation consultant was to be compared to standard care. Standard breastfeeding support within the study consisted of lactation consultant support in a BFHI-accredited hospital and breastfeeding clinic for one month. After one month, breastfeeding support is provided within the community by Child and Family Health services and lactation clinics, as well as general practitioners and private lactation consultants.

Healthy pregnant women from the local hospital were recruited and randomised into two groups, each consisting of 60 women expecting singleton births. The women were planning to deliver their infants at a local hospital. Resources for home and hospital visiting, such as a car and iPhone for text messaging, access to equipment such as nipple shields, and education resources from the postnatal ward were made available for the intervention lactation consultant to use.

I was caring for the intervention group and supported pregnant women from 37 weeks gestation until the baby was six months old, while the second group received standard care. The study was designed in consultation with researchers, postnatal hospital staff and lactation consultants, using BFHI principles and guidelines. Ethics approval was granted from the local health district prior to the commencement of the study.

Antenatal support

The first antenatal visit consisted of a visit to a venue of the mother's choice – her home, at the hospital or in a coffee shop. A suitable time was arranged for the lactation consultant and woman to meet. The birth partner was welcome to attend. An explanation of what was to be provided and what the woman could expect by having one-on-one lactation support was undertaken, with time for questions to be answered at the end. The mother was given a business card with my contact details and invited to phone or text message me at any time.

A medical and surgical history was undertaken, including an examination of the women's breasts and nipples if the mother had any concerns, for example flat or inverted nipples. As any scarring on the breast may cause breastfeeding problems, it was important to know if the mother had undergone breast surgery, such as breast implants or a breast reduction.

Education was given to prepare the mother for what was to come after birth and expect when in hospital. The importance of skin-to-skin contact and the first feed within the first hour following birth, or initiating expression of breastmilk if the baby was unable to suck for any reason, was discussed.

Antenatal expressing was commenced twice a day for five minutes, following permission from the obstetric team. Equipment was supplied to the mother, as well as a short video from the United Kingdom BFHI website on hand expressing.

By practising antenatal hand expressing before the baby was born, the mother gained confidence and learned a worthwhile skill to use after the birth, if she could not breastfeed because of sore nipples or if she was separated from her baby. Learning to express during the antenatal period also provided varying amounts of antenatal milk, which was stored and available if required later.

Some mothers are anxious because they cannot visualise how much milk their infant is getting when breastfeeding. Normal breastmilk production increases and changes over the first few days following birth, and when the baby stimulates the breasts by sucking and feeding the milk supply is increased. As the baby moves from placental feeding to breastfeeding, their stomach stretches as the volumes increase. The small amounts of colostrum, which is thick and creamy in the beginning and similar to amniotic fluid swallowed in utero, changes to an increased amount of watery fluid milk at around day three or four post birth.

There was an in-depth discussion about recognising a good latch and nutritive sucking using visual aids (doll and breast, smaller to larger marbles to demonstrate stomach size). The Australian Breastfeeding Association Elimination chart was given to all of the intervention group women. The chart explains what is normal infant output in the first five days following birth when an infant is breastfed (see Figure 11.1).

Figure 11.1: The Australian Breastfeeding Association elimination chart

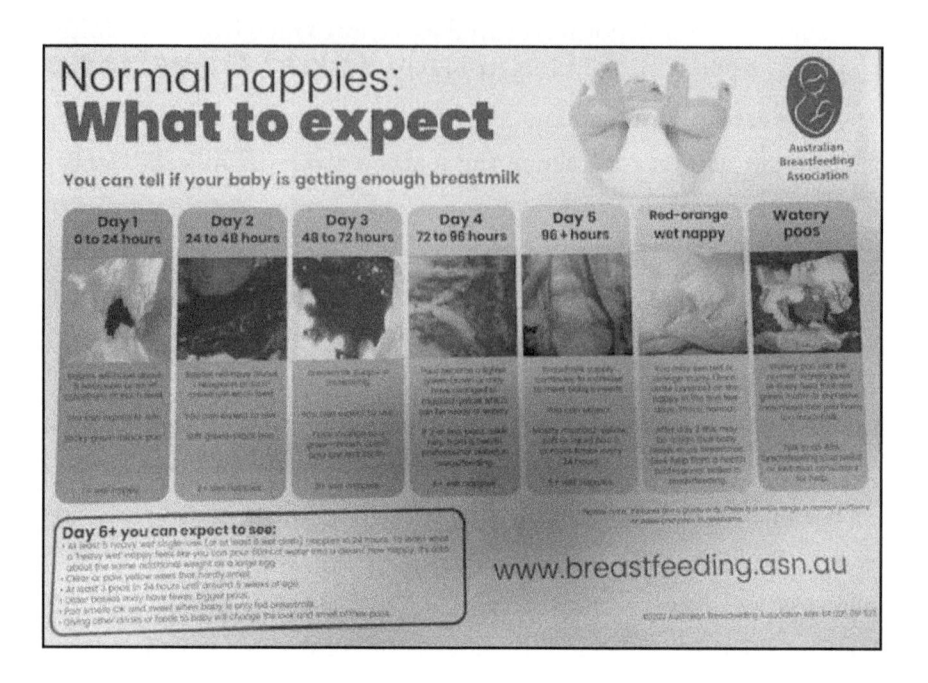

The elimination chart shows clearly the number of wet nappies and the colour of infant poos throughout the first week, and makes it easy for parents to see if their baby is being adequately hydrated. One wet nappy and the black tarry meconium poo is normal on the first day of birth. If the mother was given intravenous fluids, this may cause two or three more wet nappies within the first 24 to 48 hours following birth. If the parents observe a good latch, nutritive sucking and swallowing, while monitoring the infant's output and weight, they will come to recognise what is normal healthy growth.

Postnatal support

After the birth, a visit in hospital or at home was undertaken at the invitation of the mother. I would arrange a time with the mother when she would be feeding the baby to ensure that the latch and mother's comfort was adequate. All babies in the study received skin-to-skin contact following birth and some babies' breastfed. As a high percentage of the women who remained in hospital had a caesarean section, their infants showed little interest in sucking in the first 24 to 48 hours. Some of these infants were gagging mucus and needed time before being ready to feed and skin-to-skin contact was encouraged.

The mothers hand expressed and used the electric pump for stimulation of the breast. Because colostrum is sticky and thick, hand expressing gets more milk than electric pumping in the beginning. Available colostrum could be fed to the baby by finger, spoon or cup. The electric pump provided stimulation of the breasts to enhance milk supply. The mothers were encouraged to breastfeed when the baby showed feeding cues. Assistance with latch was given whenever the mothers requested it, as some women had tender and damaged nipples.

Antenatal expressed milk was given to the baby if an inadequate amount of freshly expressed breastmilk was not available, the infant did not feed or the mother had no other milk. Some babies were jaundiced or had low blood sugars and required more milk. These mothers were assisted with breastfeeding and cup feeding of expressed milk, or commercial baby milk if the mother's own milk was unavailable. Ensuring a sleepy baby has adequate milk and is well hydrated is important, as fluids help eliminate the high bilirubin levels that cause jaundice.

Some mothers who had a medical condition, such as diabetes or a heavy blood loss during labour, had a delay in the onset of milk production. Several of the women in the study required extra breastfeeding support due to these issues. Commercial baby milk was used when no breastmilk was available. A baby with low blood sugars or high bilirubin levels are sound medical reasons for the use of commercial baby milk.

The mother, partner and family were given a demonstration of how to set up an electric pump to encourage help from family members, as well as education on why supporting new mothers is important. A referral was made within the hospital lactation service to ensure that any women with underlying issues were known to the service.

Post-hospital care

During the hospital stay and following hospital discharge, the women received lactation support visits when requested. I contacted the women regularly by text to offer help. Text messaging was the preferred communication when women wanted an issue clarified or a problem addressed. Calls and visits were made for women with feeding problems, such as engorgement, blocked ducts, difficulties with latch and nipple pain. Anxious first-time parents with unsettled infants received extra encouragement and reassurance about normal infant behaviour, as well as demonstrations of bathing, safe sleeping and keeping their infant cool within the summer months.

Some infants had slow weight gain and required referral to their general practitioner for follow up. Two women had retained placental products, which causes a reduced milk supply and infection, while several other women had complications such as mastitis or a wound infection. Once the problems were treated and extra lactation support given, milk supply increased and the babies gained weight and continued to breastfeed.

Support groups

When the babies were around six weeks old, mothers were divided into groups of ten and invited to a morning tea to set up mother-to-mother support meetings. COVID immunisation was mandatory to attend.

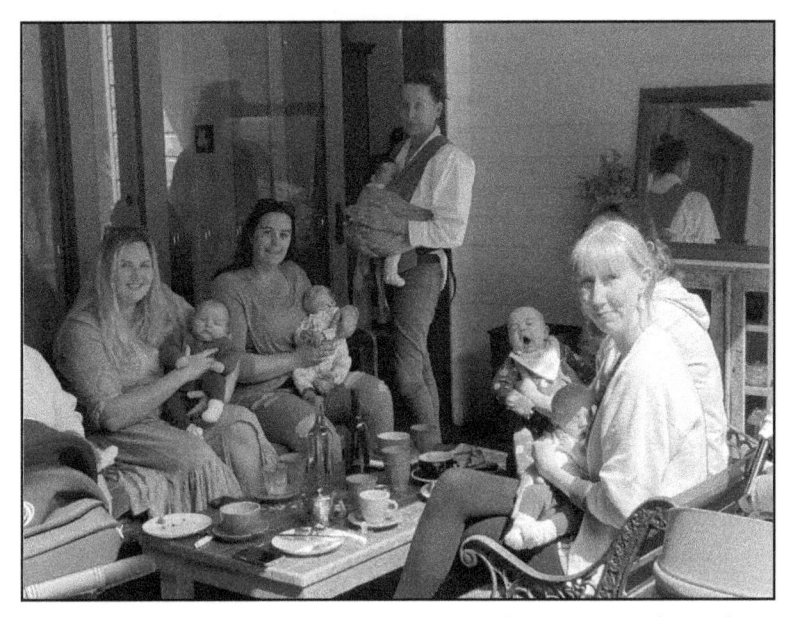

An EQUIP mother's group morning tea (Media permission obtained)

At the meetings, the mothers set up social media pages and organised group chats and social events. The first morning tea was held in my home and was followed by meetings at a local coffee shop. These meetings were ongoing, with shared baby activities once the COVID lockdowns eased such as the local library baby and toddler programs, baby music, and swimming and movie mornings. Some mothers raised the topic of when to introduce a bottle as a way of including their partner or family member in newborn care. In these situations it was important to clarify if the mother was really saying she wanted to bottle feed or needed more help. Discussions occurred within the mother's group and the women supported each other while appropriate education was given on supply and demand of breastmilk production. Discussions about other ways to include the partner or family member when caring for a baby included the importance of skin-to-skin contact with both parents, bathing, walks, play, settling and nappy changing.

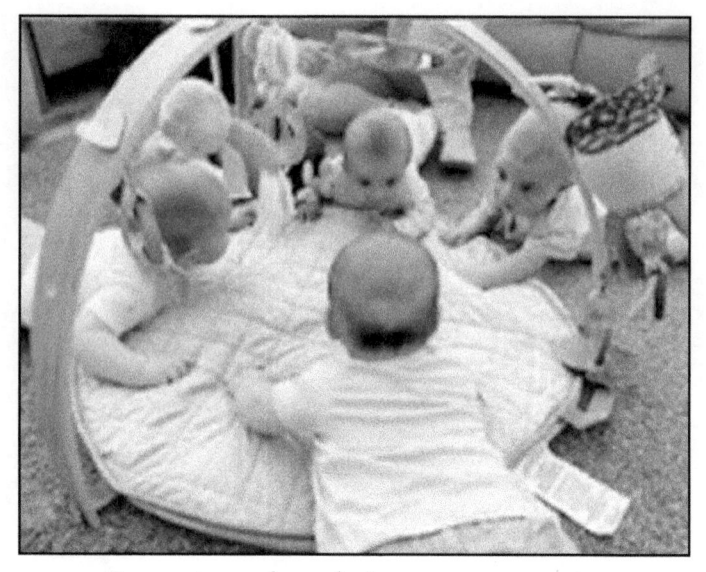

Tummy time at the mother's support group meeting

Six months' support

I ensured that all mothers had ongoing support, text messaging them at least once a week until their babies were around six months of age to check that they were going well. At that stage parents were encouraged to introduce appropriate family foods while continuing to breastfeed. Education and literature were supplied at this time. Mothers were also given information if required on breastfeeding when returning to work, and their rights in the workplace and community.

I remain in contact with many of the mothers, who have provided invaluable support to other new mothers and babies. One mother told me that she would like to pay the care she received forward when I told her of a new mother who was relocating to her suburb from Sydney. She said she would give her a call and link her in with other local mothers.

The evaluated data for the research study is not yet available. However, from the already completed and analysed data the research team leader has told me the main differences between the two groups come from the comments of the mothers. She said that although the breastfeeding rates were higher when the babies were four months of age in the continuity of care group, the women also said they felt well supported. The project manager told me that the comments from the standard care group made for heartbreaking reading and analysis, with many of the women saying they struggled alone and had to tough it out, particularly during COVID-19.

Different models of postnatal support

When women leave hospital following birth, breastfeeding may not have been established. As the randomised control trial showed, it is during this period of time women need correct information and practical support. I made many home visits during those early days because of latching issues, nipple pain, damage and engorgement of the breasts, and sleepy or difficult to feed infants. Most women find it hard to think when they are tired and lack support and, without correct information, commercial baby milk, a bottle with breastmilk, or a dummy may be introduced. New mothers are not meant to be left alone to care for a baby. I found that I was welcomed into the homes of my 60 women as an extra pair of hands with practical support and time to give.

Previous International and Australian studies have demonstrated how breastfeeding rates can be improved by well-targeted support. In 2005, researchers in the United States showed breastfeeding rates were improved (53.0 per cent vs 39.3 per cent) in a randomised control trial when the intervention group of Hispanic and Black women from the Bronx were offered individualised, prenatal and postnatal lactation support for one year compared to standard care (Bonuck et al, 2005). Three hundred and four participants were compared (intervention: n = 145; control: n = 159). The lactation consultants attempted two prenatal meetings, a postpartum hospital visit and/or home visits and telephone calls.

In Sweden in 2010, when breastfeeding women and midwives with breastfeeding knowledge and experience were interviewed, the content analysis showed that individualised breastfeeding support increases confidence and satisfaction (Bäckström et al, 2010). In order to feel confident in their new motherhood role, the women wanted more confirmation as unique individuals and as breastfeeding women. They wanted to be listened to, and they wanted more time, understanding and follow-up from health professionals.

In Australia in 2011, when researchers investigated women's perceptions and experiences of breastfeeding support, they concluded, 'Organisational systems and services that facilitate continuity of caregiver, for example continuity of midwifery care or peer support models, are more likely to facilitate an authentic presence, involving supportive care and a trusting relationship with professionals' (Schmied et al, 2011).

In Hong Kong, researchers compared 722 first-time mothers in a three-armed randomised control trial (Fu et al, 2014). The interventions were (1) standard postnatal maternity care, (2) standard care plus three 30 to 45-minute in-hospital professional breastfeeding support, or (3) standard care plus weekly 20 to 30-minute post-discharge breastfeeding telephone support for four weeks. The results demonstrated any and exclusive breastfeeding rates were higher when breastfeeding women received extra support (Fu et al, 2014).

There is ample evidence that women have been dissatisfied with postnatal hospital care and breastfeeding support for decades, and copious research shows how breastfeeding care can be improved. In some studies women describe professional support unfavourably, citing time pressures, lack of availability or guidance, promotion of unhelpful practices and conflicting advice. Midwives' support in maternity wards has been proven to impact women's breastfeeding experiences and yet misogynistic and outdated attitudes continue to prevail.

12

Discussion and Conclusion

When I began putting my thoughts into words, I wanted answers to questions I had pondered on for years. What is it that makes a mother? And how can we make life better for mothering women? What is it that gives women the resilience to persevere with breastfeeding? Many women have told me they loved breastfeeding after the initial learning phase and were sad when they stopped.

I am an elder and ready to retire. I am speaking out because, in Australia, the lives of new mothers and babies have not improved over a long period of time. Hospitals and university-affiliated maternity units in Australia were originally set up in the nineteenth and early twentieth centuries by an elite of dominant, well-educated white men, who used their power base within society to subordinate independent midwives and birthing women. These obstetricians silenced those who questioned their authority using the mantra 'healthy mother, healthy baby' without paying attention to the woman's long-term mental and physical health and the end goal of mothering.

In Australia, in 2023, the National Core Maternity Indicators reported that in 2021, 38 per cent of all women giving birth in Australia had a caesarean section and 33 per cent were first-time mothers (Australian Institute of Health and Welfare, 2023b). Research from the United States examining the postnatal health of employed women at five weeks post birth, demonstrated caesarean section was associated with significantly worse physical function, role limitation and vitality, and indicated a need for ongoing rest and recovery. The researchers concluded that the progressively growing practice of caesarean deliveries needed to be reassessed by the medical community (McGovern et al, 2006). After controlling for socio-economic conditions, a study in 2015 found when analysing relevant morbidity outcomes at a population level that caesarean section rates higher than around 10 per cent were not associated with substantial decreases in maternal and neonatal mortality. Higher caesarean section rates may not be necessary to achieve the lowest maternal and neonatal mortality rates at the population level (Ye et al, 2016).

In a recent report from the WHO monitoring the statistics of the SDGs, the authors stated, 'Pregnancy, childbirth and the postnatal period should bring positive experiences, ensuring that women and their babies reach their full potential for health and wellbeing. Although important progress has been made in the last two decades, about 287,000 women died during and following pregnancy and childbirth in 2020 (WHO, 2024b).

Physical and emotional wellbeing following birth is an integral component when becoming a mother. Birthing and breastfeeding are hard, and if a nation and community want positive mothering and healthy and bright children, families need to be supported with best practices to achieve optimum outcomes. WHO states, 'All women need access to high-quality care in pregnancy and during and after child-birth. It is particularly important that all pregnant women receive adequate antenatal care, and that all births are attended by skilled health professionals. To improve maternal health, barriers that limit access to quality maternal health services must be identified and addressed at both health system and societal levels' (WHO, 2024a).

To research this book, I travelled widely to seek knowledge. Scandinavian countries such as Norway and Denmark lead the world in terms of rights for women and families, using monies from sovereign wealth funds for the betterment of society. Women are not excluded from education and supported when having children and returning to work.

When visiting Japan, I travelled throughout the country, listening to leaders within the maternal and child health fields where community-based family support structures to address the deleterious impacts of Japan's low birth rate and isolation of women had been introduced. In travelling with a group of midwives, including Indigenous midwives, to the Northern Territory, I learned from the midwives and women within the hospitals and communities of the maternity practices that nurture mothering and are serious women's business. The elder women with the knowledge support their young mothers where ancient laws expect Indigenous women to protect their young. We also learned how the Indigenous culture of Australia has practised sustainable caring of the country for thousands of years. Since colonisation, the First Nations people have been pushed to the margins. All Australians would be better served if Australia was a more inclusive society and allowed Indigenous people to share their knowledge, while Indigenous Australians would benefit from scientific and health knowledge to improve their health and life expectancy rates.

The current bias towards medicalised birth and commercial baby milk products has had a negative impact on women and infants. Society needs to consider how the unnecessary use of both medicalised birth and commercial baby milk disempowers women as mothers. Both take away from women's autonomy and leave women with long-term emotional and physical scars. Birth is not meant to occur at a convenient time for the doctor or hospital, and commercial baby milk is a deviation from normal. While there are times when both caesarean section and commercial infant milk is appropriate, the current high intervention rates are causing harm.

Most men want their families to be heathy and well provided for. Healthy mothers improve the lives of their infants and family.

When caring for new mothers most partners will support whatever decision she makes. However, I have seen fathers agree to their baby receiving commercial baby milk after being asked by NICU staff when the mother is unavailable (she maybe still in the operating theatre), only to find the mother angry and undermined because she was not included in the decision. Health professionals need to be mindful when providing information to families and use evidence-based information.

Oxytocin-inducing care behaviours reduce stress and enhance bonding and protective behaviours in parents. One such behaviour was made public in a report from the WHO in 2023. In Vietnam, 'an early essential newborn care (EENC) initiative to promote a "first embrace" after caesarean section was shown to save babies lives. Due to an increasing number of caesarean sections in Vietnam (29 per cent nationally in 2022), neonatal intensive care nurseries (NICUs) became overcrowded because all caesarean section born infants were sent to NICU for prolonged observation. This caused an increased risk in newborn infections and other complications, including the introduction of commercial infant baby milk. The package of evidence-based interventions with non-separation of the mother and infant at the core included immediate and thorough drying of the infant, sustained skin-to-skin contact of the mother and baby, delayed cord clamping, promotion of early and exclusive breastfeeding, resuscitation of non-breathing babies and 'kangaroo mother care'. At the Da Nang Hospital for Women and Children, data from 16,927 newborns delivered by caesarean section between 2013 and 2015 — before and after the introduction of the intervention – was collected and demonstrated a decrease in the total number of NICU admissions from 16.7 per cent to 11.8 per cent. In addition, compared with the pre-intervention period, the number of babies with hypothermia on admission to the NICU declined from 5.0 per cent to 3.7 per cent and cases of sepsis decreased from 3.2 per cent to 0.8 per cent. Prior to the intervention, more than half of all newborns in the NICU were fed something other than breastmilk. After the package was introduced, 85.8 per cent of infants were exclusively breastfed and preterm newborns (< 2000 g) receiving KMC increased from 50 per cent to 67 per cent. The reduction in caesarean NICU admissions also represented a cost saving to the hospital of at least US$162,060 in the year after introducing the intervention and led to the early essential newborn care package being adopted widely throughout Vietnam'.(WHO, 2021)

My story: Stress and breastfeeding

I am still in contact with a mother of 18-year-old triplet girls. Following caesarean section she was separated from her infants. She saw the babies fleetingly when they were born before they were taken to the neonatal intensive care unit and she was transferred to the postnatal ward. I was the midwife caring for the mother the morning following the birth and found her very stressed. I could see she had no interest in anything other than being reunited with her babies. I prioritised her care to enable a visit to the NICU as soon as possible. Once she was with her infants and the stress hormones were reduced, we were able to go about the business of hand expressing colostrum to feed the babies. Colostrum protects an infant's gut lining from infection and increases blood sugar levels without the need for commercial baby milk, and is extremely important for low-birth-weight babies such as her triplets. Stress hormones inhibit breastmilk production. The mother recognised and stopped me at the local supermarket checkout queue seven years after the babies were born. She told me that she had always wanted to say thank you as at the time all that mattered to her was being with her infants and I had recognised her distress at being separated from them.

****

In the past many midwives, including myself, have been belittled as non-scientific by other health professionals when promoting caring behaviours. While having had a baby or struggling to breastfeed is not a prerequisite for being either an obstetrician or a midwife, having walked in the woman's shoes does make it easier to empathise with women.

If given the opportunity with time and supportive staff, new mothers can learn. Some mothers may be frightened or not ready or have never held a baby, while others may be revisited by past trauma such as a difficult breastfeeding experience or history of abuse. Others may be in pain or under the influence of medications.

The physicians who influenced birth and infant feeding within the English colonies came from an elite whose theories were based on little evidence with breastfeeding mothers and work with motherless children. When I became a nurse and midwife, I learned and accepted the lessons from the institutional-based education, but as a mother I instinctively questioned some practices. For example, when a hospital-based, family birth centre and midwifery-led model of care was being introduced and challenged by the status quo, I promoted the facility amongst my daughters and friends. My experience had taught me that all mothers do not need the medicalised model. My daughters, like their grandmothers before them, were healthy young women with no risk factors. I encouraged them to trust themselves in the safety of competent midwives within the birthing centre close to hospital services. My daughters had normal births, leaving the birthing centres to return home with healthy infants within several hours of birth and minimal interventions, and breastfed to WHO recommendations. I know this is not possible for all women, however I also know the risks posed to women due to the current capitalist system.

Historically since colonisation, and today, some conservative members of society within the Capitalist model continue to exploit and abuse women both physically and emotionally. Rather than recognising women as equal members of society with gender-specific attributes that nurture and make society healthier and kinder, women are undermined, particularly when vulnerable following birth and during breastfeeding. As the Australian breastfeeding report card into policies and programs that improve breastfeeding rates issued by the World Breastfeeding Trends Initiative demonstrates, Australia has failed. Without greater improvements from 25.5/100 in 2017 to 33/100 in 2023, Australian breastfeeding rates will not reach Sustainable Development Goal targets (see Figure 12.1).

Figure 12.1: Breastfeeding Trends Initiative report card, 2023

WBTi
World Breastfeeding Trends Initiative (WBTi)

Australia: Report Card 2023 — 33/100

The assessment of implementation of policies and programs from the World Health Organization's Global Strategy for Infant and Young Child Feeding (GSIYCF).

Policies and programs: Indicators 1–10

IBFAN Asia Guidelines for WBTi for rating individual indicators 1 to 15 are as follows: 0–3 is rated Red, 4–6 is rated Yellow, 7–9 is rated Blue and more than 9 is rated Green.

#	Indicator	Score out of 10
1.	**National Policy, Governance and Funding** — Concerns national policy, plan of action, funding and coordination issues.	1.5
2.	**Baby Friendly Hospital Initiative / Ten Steps to Successful Breastfeeding** — Concerns percentage BFHI hospitals, training, standard monitoring, assessment and reassessment systems.	6
3.	**Implementation of the International Code of Marketing of Breastmilk Substitutes (WHO Code) and all subsequent World Health Assembly (WHA) Resolutions** — Concerns implementation of the Code as law, monitored and enforced.	5
4.	**Maternity protection** — Concerns paid maternity leave, paid breastfeeding breaks, national legislation encouraging workplace accommodation for breastfeeding and/or childcare and ratification of ILO MPC No 183.	6
5.	**Health and Nutrition Care Systems (in support of breastfeeding & IYCF)** — Concerns health provider schools and pre-service education programs, standards and guidelines for mother-friendly childbirth procedures and in-service training programs.	2.5
6.	**Counselling Services for Pregnant and Breastfeeding Mothers** — Concerns the availability of and women's access to skilled counselling services on infant and young child feeding during pregnancy and after childbirth.	6
7.	**Accurate and Unbiased Information Support** — Concerns public education and communication strategy for improving infant and young child feeding that is actively implemented at local levels.	2
8.	**Infant Feeding and HIV** — Concerns policy and programs to address infant feeding and HIV issue and on-going monitoring of the effects of interventions on infant feeding practices and health outcomes for mothers and infants.	4
9.	**Infant and young child feeding during emergencies (IYCF-E)** — Concerns policy and program on IYCF-E and material on IYCF-E integrated into pre-service and in-service training for emergency management.	0
10.	**Monitoring and Evaluation** — Concerns monitoring, management and information systems as part of the planning and management process.	0

Subtotal: 33/100

Feeding practices: Indicators 11–15

Requires national data that is no more than five years old and meets the WHO indicators for assessing IYCF practices.

Indicator	Data	Score out of 10
Initiation of Breastfeeding (within 1 hour)	No available data	0/10
Exclusive Breastfeeding under 6 months	No available data	0/10
Median duration of breastfeeding	No available data	0/10
Bottle-feeding (0-12 months)	No available data	0/10
Complementary Feeding (6-8 months)	No available data	0/10
Subtotal		0/50

Total score = 33/100

The full report is available at www.wbtiaus.com or wbtiaus@gmail.com

Australia: Report Card 2023

Gaps	Recommendations
There is no effective implementation of The International Code of Marketing of Breast-milk Substitutes and subsequent World Health Assembly resolutions have not been adopted or implemented in full.	All Australian governments should fully implement the International Code and fund its monitoring and enforcement free from commercial influence to ensure full compliance including in the health system.
The International Code is not effectively implemented and there is nothing to prevent commercial influence on policy.	
Australian jurisdictions have not implemented Baby Friendly Health Initiative (BFHI) in the health system due in part to inadequate funding. This means health professionals are inadequately prepared for supporting breastfeeding women and their babies. The Australian National Breastfeeding Strategy (ANBS) 2019 priority action areas (including BFHI) do not have specific funding allocated.	Include funding for BFHI in all state and jurisdictions to implement BFHI accreditation in the National Health Reform Agreement. The implementation of the ANBS should be included in the meeting agenda for Australian health ministers at least twice a year.
Australian breastfeeding targets stated in the ANBS and the NHMRC Infant Feeding Guidelines are not consistent with the infant and young child feeding practices recommended by the World Health Organization (WHO) regarding duration of exclusive and continued breastfeeding. Nor are FSANZ food standards for packaging and labelling of baby foods.	Update the NHMRC Dietary guidelines to • align fully with WHO breastfeeding recommendations, • include detailed guidance for health workers on supporting breastfeeding in emergencies and disasters, • update recommendations in line with recent evidence to protect all women's rights to breastfeed regardless of HIV status, child protection status or incarceration. Align baby food labelling to align with WHO recommendations of exclusive breastfeeding for 6 months.
The monitoring and reporting requirements in the ANBS have not been actioned.	Revise the ANBS implementation and timelines and make these publicly available.
The baseline evaluation due in July 2019-June 2020 was not funded or actioned.	Fund a Australian National Infant Feeding Survey, a Priority Action in the ANBS at least every five years.
There is no nationally consistent collection of quality data that monitors the effectiveness of the ANBS or how infants and young children are fed.	

Core Group Members

Naomi Hull BN BN Grad. Cert. Nursing, Cert IV Breastfeeding Ed (Counselling), IBCLC, MPH

Julie Smith BEc (Hons)/B A (Asian Studies), PhD, Cert IV Breastfeeding Ed (Counselling) Cert IV Breastfeeding Ed (Community)

Jen Hocking RN RM BA BN Grad Dip Mid MMid PhD

Libby Salmon BVSc MVS Cert IV Breastfeeding Ed (Counselling)

Susan Tawia BSc, PhD, Cert IV Breastfeeding Ed (Community), Dip Breastfeeding Management

Decalie Brown RN CM CFHN BHNg FILCA IBCLC

Karleen Gribble BRurSc (Hons), PhD, Cert IV Breastfeeding Ed. (Community and Counselling).

Helen Adams RM IBCLC

Heather Gale RN RM IBCLC Post-graduate Diploma Nurse Education, Master of Nursing, (Former Breastfeeding Counsellor, Australian Breastfeeding Association).

Tracey Foster DipHSc Grad Dip Mid IBCLC CFHN Grad Dip Mgmt Grad Cert IV in Assessment & Workplace Training, Grad Cert Clinical Teaching

Elaine Burns RM, RN, BN, MCN(Midwifery), PhD

Bindi Borg PhD, M. International and Community Development, MA, BA, Cert IV Breastfeeding Education (Counselling and Community), Cert IV (Training and Assessment)

List of the partners for the assessment process

Core group
- Australian Breastfeeding Association
- Lactation Consultants of Australia and New Zealand

Reference Group
- Breastfeeding Coalition Tasmania
- Maternal Child and Family Health Nurses Australia (MCaFHNA)

Individuals
- Mary-Anne Land PhD, MPH
- Nina Chad PhD
- Professor Lisa Amir, MBBS MMed PhD IBCLC
- Kathleen Halliday AdvAPD, IBCLC

IBFAN   WBTi

The World Breastfeeding Trends Initiative (WBTi) is IBFAN Asia's flagship. WBTi is being implemented as an integral part of two projects "Global Breastfeeding Initiative for Child Survival" (GBICS), in partnership with the Norwegian Agency for Development Cooperation (Norad) and Global Proposal for Coordinated Action of IBFAN and WABA Protecting, Promoting and Supporting Breastfeeding through Human Rights and Gender Equality" in partnership with Swedish International Development Agency (Sida).

The history of Australia since 1788 has created ongoing rules, which benefit an elite and exploit others due to hierarchical power structures. It is the unequal distribution of resources that creates inequity and brings society into conflict. The patriarchal ideas of the past have led religion to harness the biology of women to benefit the capitalist model, and the lack of progress that leads to the premature death of many women and children across the world comes about because of a patriarchal male elite and a greedy economic system.

Most Australian women do not commence a family until their thirties. Leaving the workforce to have children leaves women disadvantaged. In an article published in *The Guardian* for International Women's Day in 2023, Greg Jericho reported that Australian women earn $1 million less on average over their lifetime than men and retire with $136,000 less in superannuation. The same article reported that the Association of Superannuation Funds of Australia estimated that women earning a median wage would accumulate $393,676 in super earnings, $151,000 below the level defined as a 'comfortable retirement'. Why should this be so?

The SDG statistical report states that the targets to be achieved by 2030 have markedly stalled since 2015, and that it will be challenging to achieve the targets by 2030. The second of five key areas for urgent action requires governments to advance concrete, integrated and targeted policies and actions to eradicate poverty, reduce inequality and end the war on nature, with a focus on advancing the rights of women and girls and empowering the most vulnerable (WHO, 2023a, 2023b).

The Federal Office for Women is ideally suited to bring about changes for women using the SDG targets and infant feeding resources as a way forward. The science demonstrates breastfeeding is best for the mother, baby, environment and the economy. Australia has a Breastfeeding Strategy and requires an Australian co-ordinator with appropriate authority, resources and multisector participation for the strategy to be implemented.

Since the Second World War, families who survived and set about rebuilding their lives in the suburbs now see their children and grandchildren unable to afford a family and home. Young couples are struggling to pay off an education debt and are leaving the luxury of having a family until they can house themselves. Migration has been used as a prop to support Australia's otherwise failing population levels, workforce and economy, and one quarter of new mothers are vulnerable migrant women.

After a lifetime of working with newly birthed mothers, I have come to the conclusion that without solid structural changes that support women and recognise their valuable contribution as partners within society, many women will either have no children or have insufficient children to maintain population replacement levels. Women are vulnerable when having a baby and make a physical, emotional and financial sacrifice, which ultimately benefits all of society, and they should be nurtured. Mothers evolve with positive role models within their own families and society and vice versa. We copy what we have learnt. There is an urgent need for Human Rights legislation reform to protect all Australians which includes women during maternity to support them to bring up healthy, well-educated children who, in turn, will underpin the wellbeing and economy of the nation.

I am not interested in getting into the breast-versus-bottle debate, which has been used to divide women and nurses for decades. Some women choose not to breastfeed, and that is their choice. Some women do not breastfeed because they have underlying issues. However, the majority of women can breastfeed if they are given timely, accurate information and support. Unfortunately, rather than blame an unsupportive system or greedy economic model, I think lateral or horizontal violence occurs. Lateral violence occurs within marginalised groups, with members striking out at each other as a result of being oppressed. The oppressed become the oppressors of themselves and each other. Bullying, name calling, backstabbing are common behaviours that prevent positive change.

There is considerable evidence from Professor Amy Brown, Director of the Centre for Lactation, Infant Feeding and Translation at Swansea University, demonstrating women experience grief when unable to achieve their breastfeeding goals (Brown, 2018). I have supported many women to breastfeed and believe, if supported and given the best available care, woman are not angry when they are unable to breastfeed. They may be sad as are women who have to leave their infants in the care of others for economic reasons, but they do not feel the same anger or frustration or grief as women left to struggle alone feel.

One supporter of a petition to the Australian Parliament for a Medicare rebate for lactation consultants gave her reason for signing the petition as 'Breastfeeding is the last bastion of hope'. I am of a similar mind and believe breastfeeding provides the foundational building blocks for the health and wellbeing of families, and the environment.

References

Akre, James (2016) 'Breastfeeding: One Man's Perspective', Huffpost, 12 May 2016, https://www.huffpost.com/entry/breastfeeding-one-mans-perspective_b_57343d70e4b0ed0ca07a7cb3. Accessed 3 July 2024.

Almeida HCCD, Candido LKD, Harrison D, Bueno M (2018) 'Be Sweet to Babies: evaluation of an instructional video on neonatal pain management by nurses', *Revista da Escola de Enfermagem da USP*, 52, p. e03313.

Almroth SG (1978) 'Water requirements of breast-fed infants in a hot climate', *The American Journal of Clinical Nutrition* 31(7), pp1 154–1157.

Australasian Health Infrastructure Alliance (2023) *Australasian Health Facility Guidelines – Maternity Units*, https://www.hinfra.health.nsw.gov.au/news/latest/latest/updated-aushfg-guidance-for-maternity-units. Accessed 24 June 2024.

Australian Bureau of Statistics (2021) *Births, Australia*, <https://www.abs.gov.au/statistics/people/population/births-australia/2021>. Accessed 30 June 2024.

Australian College of Midwives (2018), 'bfhi_information_for_maternity_facilities_20170830.pdf'. Accessed 3 July 2024.

Australian Institute of Health and Welfare (2023a) *Australia's mothers and babies* report AIHW, Australian Government, https://www.aihw.gov.au/reports/mothers-babies/australias-mothers-babies/contents/about. Accessed 10 June 2024.

Australian Institute of Health and Welfare (2023b) *National Core Maternity Indicators* report, https://www.aihw.gov.au/reports/mothers-babies/national-core-maternity-indicators/contents/summary-1. Accessed 9 June 2024.

Bäckström CA, Wahn EI, Ekström AC (2010) 'Two sides of breastfeeding support: experiences of women and midwives', *Int Breastfeed J*. Nov 29;5:20. doi: 10.1186/1746-4358-5-20. PMID: 21114812; PMCID: PMC3001698.

Barnard J and Twigg K (2014) *Nursing Mums: A History of the Australian Breastfeeding Association 1964–2014*, Australian Breastfeeding Association, Victoria.

Beake S, Bick D, Narracott C, Chang YS (2017) 'Interventions for women who have a caesarean birth to increase uptake and duration of breastfeeding: A systematic review', *Matern Child Nutr*, Oct;13(4):e12390. doi: 10.1111/mcn.12390. Epub 2016 Nov 24. PMID: 27882659; PMCID: PMC6866035.

Bergman NJ (2019a) 'Birth practices: Maternal-neonate separation as a source of toxic stress', Birth Defects Res, Sep 1;111(15):1087-1109. doi: 10.1002/bdr2.1530. Epub 2019 Jun 3. PMID: 31157520.

Bergman NJ (2019b) 'Historical background to maternal-neonate separation and neonatal care', *Birth Defects Res*, Sep 1;111(15):1081–1086. doi: 10.1002/bdr2.1528. Epub 2019 May 30. PMID: 31148388.

Bergman NJ, Carney G, Ludington-Hoe SM (2010) 'Kangaroo care for the preterm infant', ICAN: Infant, *Child & Adolescent Nutrition*, 2(3), pp 165–169.

Bergman NJ, Linley LL, Fawcus SR (2004) 'Randomized controlled trial of skin-to-skin contact from birth versus conventional incubator for physiological stabilization in 1200- to 2199-gram newborns', *Acta paediatrica*, Oslo, Norway: 1992, 93(6), 779–785.

Betrán AP, Ye J, Moller AB, Zhang J, Gülmezoglu AM, Torloni MR (2016) 'The Increasing Trend in Caesarean Section Rates: Global, Regional and National Estimates: 1990-2014', *PLoS One*, Feb 5;11(2):e0148343. doi: 10.1371/journal.pone.0148343. PMID: 26849801; PMCID: PMC4743929.

Bonuck KA, Trombley M, Freeman K, McKee D (2005) 'Randomized, controlled trial of a prenatal and postnatal lactation consultant intervention on duration and intensity of breastfeeding up to 12 months', *Pediatrics*, Dec 116(6):1413-26. doi: 10.1542/peds.2005-0435. PMID: 16322166.

Brodribb W, Fallon AB, Jackson C, Hegney D (2009) 'Breastfeeding knowledge: the experiences of Australian general practice registrars', *Australian Family Physician* 38, no. ½, 26–29.

Brown A (2018) 'What do women lose if they are prevented from meeting their breastfeeding goals?', *Clinical Lactation*, 9(4), pp 200–207.

Bystrova K, Ivanova V, Edhborg M, Matthiesen AS, Ransjö-Arvidson AB, Mukhamedrakhimov R, Uvnäs-Moberg K, Widström AM (2009) 'Early contact versus separation: effects on mother-infant interaction one year later', *Birth* Jun 36(2):97–109. doi: 10.1111/j.1523-536X.2009.00307.x. PMID: 19489802.

Cai Y and Feng W (2021) 'The social and sociological consequences of China's one-child policy', *Annual Review of Sociology*, 47(1), pp 587–606.

Centre for Epidemiology and Evidence (2022), HealthStats NSW, Ministry of Health, https://www.healthstats.nsw.gov.au/r/113833. Accessed 3 July 2024.

Chan GJ, Valsangkar B, Kajeepeta S, Boundy EO, Wall S (2016) 'What is kangaroo mother care? Systematic review of the literature', Journal of Global Health, 6(1).

Clun R and Thomson A (2023) 'The people whose life choices will shape Australia for the next decade', Sydney Morning Herald.

COAG Health Council (2019) *The Australian National Breastfeeding Strategy: 2019 and Beyond*, Department of Health, Canberra.

Colaizy TT, Bartick MC, Jegier BJ, et al. Impact of Optimized Breastfeeding on the Costs of Necrotizing Enterocolitis in Extremely Low Birthweight Infants. *J Pediatr*. 2016;175:100-105. e2. doi:10.1016/j.jpeds.2016.03.040

Commonwealth of Australia, House of Representatives Standing Committee on Health and Ageing (2009) 'Improving Maternity Services in Australia', *The Report of the Maternity Services Review*, Canberra. Accessed: 04/07/2024

Commonwealth of Australia (2007) *The Best Start: report on the inquiry into the health benefits of breastfeeding*, Commonwealth of Australia, Canberra, https://nla.gov.au/nla.obj-2177371144. Accessed 21 June 2024.

Demos, J (2008) *The Enemy Within: A Short History of Witch-hunting*, Penguin, New York.

Development Neonatal Research Network (2016) 'Impact of optimized breastfeeding on the costs of necrotizing enterocolitis in extremely low birthweight infants', *J Pediatr.* Aug;175:100–105.e2. doi: 10.1016/j.jpeds.2016.03.040. Epub Apr 27. PMID: 27131403; PMCID: PMC5274635.

Dunn PM (2007) 'Arvo Ylppö (1887–1992): pioneer of Finnish paediatrics', *Arch Dis Child Fetal Neonatal Ed.*, May 92(3):F230–2. doi: 10.1136/adc.2005.077552. PMID: 17449859; PMCID: PMC2675334.

Epstein-Gilboa K (2006) 'Systemic interactions in breastfeeding families', tspace.library.utoronto.ca. Accessed 3 July 2024.

Fahy K (2007) 'An Australian history of the subordination of midwifery', *Women Birth* Mar 20(1):25–9. doi: 10.1016/j.wombi.2006.08.003. Epub 2006 Sep 14. Erratum in: Women Birth. 2007 Sep 20(3):141. PMID: 16973426.

Filippa M, Monaci MG, Spagnuolo C, Serravalle P, Daniele R, Grandjean D (2021) 'Maternal speech decreases pain scores and increases oxytocin levels in preterm infants during painful procedures', *Sci Rep.* Aug 27 11(1):17301. doi: 10.1038/s41598-021-96840-4. PMID: 34453088; PMCID: PMC8397753.

Filippa M, Monaci MG, Spagnuolo C, Di Benedetto M, Serravalle P, Grandjean D (2023) 'Oxytocin levels increase and anxiety decreases in mothers who sing and talk to their premature Infants during a painful procedure, *Children* (Basel), Feb 9 10(2):334. doi: 10.3390/children10020334. PMID: 36832462; PMCID: PMC9955880.

Fu IC, Fong DY, Heys M, Lee IL, Sham A, Tarrant M (2014) 'Professional breastfeeding support for first-time mothers: a multicentre cluster randomised controlled trial', *BJOG*, Dec

121(13):1673-83. doi: 10.1111/1471-0528.12884. Epub 2014 May 26. PMID: 24861802.

Gabbianelli R, Bordoni L, Morano S, Calleja-Agius J, Lalor JG (2020) 'Nutri-epigenetics and gut microbiota: how birth care, bonding and breastfeeding can influence and be influenced?' *Int J Mol Sci*. Jul 16 21(14):5032. doi: 10.3390/ijms21145032. PMID: 32708742; PMCID: PMC7404045.

Garnica-Torres, Z and Dias, GB, da Silva, PJ (2024) 'A systematic review of fatherhood and kangaroo care in the NICU', *Children and Youth Services Review*, Elsevier, vol. 157(C).

Glasofer A, Donato SE, Werfel E, Galosi G, Epstein HAB, Moraca C (2022) 'The relationship between maternal fluid intake during labor and neonatal weight loss: a review of the literature', *Clinical Lactation* 13(3).

Glasper EA (2020)'Romania's Forgotten Children: Sensory Deprivation Revisited', *Comprehensive Child and Adolescent Nursing*, 43(2), 81–87, https://doi.org/10.1080/24694193.2020.1735250. Accessed July 4 2024.

Greer, Germaine (1970) *The Female Eunuch*, MacGibbon and Kee, London.

Grote V, Verduci E, Scaglioni S, Vecchi F, Contarini G, Giovannini M, Koletzko B, Agostoni C, European Childhood Obesity Project (2016) 'Breast milk composition and infant nutrient intakes during the first 12 months of life' *Eur J Clin Nutr*. Feb 70(2):250-6. doi: 10.1038/ejcn.2015.162. Epub 2015 Sep 30. PMID: 26419197.

Grym K and Borgermans L (2018a) 'Public health nurses in Finland: a life-course approach to the prevention of noncommunicable diseases: good practice brief ', No. WHO/EURO: 2018-3387-43146-60410, World Health Organization, Regional Office for Europe.

Grym K and Borgermans L (2018b) 'Public health nurses in Finland: A life-course approach to the prevention of noncommunicable diseases', Compendium of Good Practices.

Haiek LN, Hansen MN, Hannula L, Ezeonodo A. How to use the Neo-BFHI Package: Tools for self-appraisal, monitoring, the external assessment process, and education material.

Hansen K (2016) 'Breastfeeding: a smart investment in people and in economies', *Lancet*, Jan 30 387(10017):416. doi: 10.1016/S0140-6736(16)00012-X. PMID: 26869553.

Harrison D, Larocque C, Reszel J, Harrold J, Aubertin C (2017) 'Be sweet to babies during painful procedures: a pilot evaluation of a parent-targeted video', Advances in Neonatal Care, 17(5), pp 372–380.

Hector D, King L, Webb, K (20050 'Factors affecting breastfeeding practices – applying a conceptual framework', NSW Public Health Bulletin, vol 16, no 3–4, p. 53.

Hirth R, Weitkamp T, Dwivedi A (2012) 'Maternal intravenous fluids and infant weight', *Clinical Lactation*, 3(2), pp 59–63.

Holmes A (2017) Becoming mother: physiological mothering practices as art and feminist activism, Doctoral dissertation, University of Sydney.

Holt LE (1894) *The Care and Feeding of Children: A Catechism for the Use of Mothers and Children's Nurses*, D Appleton and Co, New York.

Horta BL, Loret de Mola C, Victora CG (2015) 'Breastfeeding and intelligence: a systematic review and meta-analysis', *Acta Paediatr*, Dec 104(467):14-9. doi: 10.1111/apa.13139. PMID: 26211556.

Keedle H, Peters L, Schmied V, Burns E, Keedle W, Dahlen HG (2020) 'Women's experiences of planning a vaginal birth after caesarean in different models of maternity care in Australia', *BMC Pregnancy Childbirth* 20, 381.

Kennedy, RF (1968) Remarks at the University of Kansas, 18 March 1968, John F Kennedy Presidential Library.

King, Truby (1913) Feeding and Care of Baby, Royal New Zealand Society for the Health of Women and Children, New Zealand.

Lawrence RA and Lawrence RM (2021) *Biochemistry of Human Milk in Breastfeeding*, Elsevier.

Maastrup R, Hannula L, Hansen MN, Ezeonodo A, Haiek LN (2022) 'The Baby-friendly Hospital Initiative for neonatal wards. A mini review', *Acta Paediatr*. Apr 111(4):750-755. doi: 10.1111/apa.16230. Epub 2021 Dec 29. PMID: 34932843.

Maben J (2009) 'Splendid isolation? The pros and cons of single rooms for the NHS', *Nurs Manag* (Harrow), May 16(2):18-9. doi: 10.7748/nm2009.05.16.2.18.c7010. PMID: 19485004.

Mangel L, Vanetik S, Mandel D, Marom R, Lubetzky R, Moran-Lev H (2022) 'Carbohydrate content of human milk is affected by seasonal variations: a retrospective observational study', *Journal of Perinatology*, 42(8), pp.1058–1062.

McGovern P, Dowd B, Gjerdingen D, Gross CR, Kenney S, Ukestad L, McCaffrey D, Lundberg U (2006) 'Postpartum health of employed mothers 5 weeks after childbirth', *Ann Fam Med.*, Mar-Apr 4(2):159-67. doi: 10.1370/afm.519. PMID: 16569720; PMCID: PMC1467019.

Moore ER, Bergman N, Anderson GC, Medley N (2016) 'Early skin-to-skin contact for mothers and their healthy newborn infants', *Cochrane Database Syst Rev.*, Nov 25;11(11):CD003519. doi: 10.1002/14651858.CD003519.pub4. PMID: 27885658; PMCID: PMC6464366.

Mörelius E, Brogren S, Andersson S, Alehagen S (2021) 'Fathers' experiences of feeding their extremely preterm infants in family-centred neonatal intensive care: a qualitative study', *Int Breastfeed J* 16, 46.

Neu J (2014) 'Necrotizing enterocolitis', *World Rev Nutr Diet*, 110, pp 253–263.

Neu J (2020) 'Necrotizing enterocolitis: the future', *Neonatology*, 117(2), pp 240–244.

Nightingale F (1859) Notes on Hospitals, Cambridge University Press, England. https://digital.library.upenn.edu/women/nightingale/nursing/nursing.html. Accessed 6 June 2024.

Nishigori H, Obara T, Nishigori T, Metoki H, Mizuno S, Ishikuro M, Sakurai K, Hamada H, Watanabe Z, Hoshiai T, Arima T, Nakai K, Kuriyama S, Yaegashi N; Miyagi Regional Center of Japan Environment & Children's Study Group (2020) 'Mother-to-infant bonding failure and intimate partner violence during pregnancy as risk factors for father-to-infant bonding failure at 1 month postpartum: an adjunct study of the Japan Environment and Children's Study', J Matern Fetal Neonatal Med, Aug 33(16):2789-2796. doi: 10.1080/14767058.2018.1560414. Epub 2019 Apr 15. PMID: 30563397.

Nyquist KH, Häggkvist AP, Hansen MN, Kylberg E, Frandsen AL, Maastrup R, Ezeonodo A, Hannula L, Haiek LN, Baby-Friendly Hospital Initiative Expert Group (2013) 'Expansion of the baby-friendly hospital initiative ten steps to successful breastfeeding into neonatal intensive care: expert group recommendations', *J Hum Lact*. Aug 29(3):300–9. doi: 10.1177/0890334413489775. Epub 2013 May 31. PMID: 23727630.

Ochoa TJ, Mendoza K, Carcamo C, Zegarra J, Bellomo S, Jacobs J, Cossey V (2020) 'Is mother's own milk lactoferrin intake associated with reduced neonatal sepsis, necrotizing enterocolitis, and death? *Neonatology*, 117(2):167–174. doi: 10.1159/000505663. Epub 2020 Feb 13. PMID: 32053823; PMCID: PMC7381382.

Odent M, (2009) 'The masculinisation of the birth environment', *Journal of Prenatal and Perinatal Psychology and Health*, 23(3), p. 185.

Ozrenk E and Inci SS (2008) 'The effect of seasonal variation on the composition of cow milk in Van Province, Pakistan', *Journal of nutrition*', 7(1), pp 161–164.

Palit V and Opie GF (2015) 'Breastmilk banking and the Mercy Health experience', *The Medical Journal of Australia*, 203(9), pp 357–358.

Parker MG, Stellwagen LM, Noble L, Kim JH, Poindexter BB, Puopolo KM; Section on breastfeeding, Committee on nutrition, Committee on fetus and newborn (2021) 'Promoting human milk and breastfeeding for the very low birth weight infant', *Pediatrics*, Nov 148(5):e2021054272. doi: 10.1542/peds.2021-054272. Epub 2021 Oct 11. PMID: 34635582.

Parrott ML and Edwards AM (2023) 'Reproductive Strategies and Biology of the Australasian Marsupials' in Cáceres NC, Dickman CR (eds), *American and Australasian Marsupials*, Springer, Cham. https://doi.org/10.1007/978-3-030-88800-8_37-1. Accessed 6 June 2024.

Plunket, Victoria https://www.plunket.org.nz/plunket/about-plunket/who-we-are/lady-victoria-plunket/. Accessed 26 April 2024.

Quinn EA, Diki Bista K, Childs G (2016) 'Milk at altitude: Human milk macronutrient composition in a high-altitude adapted population of Tibetans', *American Journal of Physical Anthropology*, 159(2), pp 233–243.

Rendle-Short J (1960) 'William Cadogan, Eighteenth-Century Physician', Cambridge University Press, https://www.cambridge.org/core/services/aop-cambridge-core/content/view/E9AEDB5F59C95A6CF97795D42780C76F/S0025727300025631a.pdf/william_cadogan_eighteenthcentury_physician.pdf. Accessed 26 June 2024.

Rice PL (2010) 'Rooming-in and cultural practices: choice or constraint', *Journal of Reproductive and Infant Psychology*, vol. 18, no. 1, pp. 21–32.

Robinson M, (2002) Human Rights at the Heart of Peace, City of Sydney Peace Prize Lecture, Sydney Peace Foundation. https://

sydneypeacefoundation.org.au/peace-prize-recipient/2002-mary-robinson/. Accessed 26 June 2024.

Rollins NC, Bhandari N, Hajeebhoy N, Horton S, Lutter CK, Martines JC, Piwoz, EG, Richter, LM Victora, CG, Lancet Breastfeeding Series Group (2016) 'Why invest, and what will it take to improve breastfeeding practices?', Lancet, Jan 30 doi: https://doi.org/10.1016/S0140-6736(15)01044-2. Accessed 4 July 2024.

Roosevelt E (1958) 'Where Do Human Rights Begin?' Speech delivered at the United Nations, https://ask.un.org/faq/323626. Accessed 6 June 2024.

Rubin R (1967a) 'Attainment of the maternal role: Part I, processes', *Nursing Research*, 16(3), pp 237–245.

Rubin R (1967b) Attainment of the maternal role: Part II, models and referrants', *Nursing Research*, 16(4), pp 342–346.

Scarf VL, Yu S, Viney R, Lavis L, Dahlen H, Foureur M, Homer C (2020) 'The cost of vaginal birth at home, in a birth centre or in a hospital setting in New South Wales: A micro-costing study', *Women and Birth*, 33(3), pp 286–293.

Scarf VL, Yu S, Viney R, Cheah SL, Dahlen H, Sibbritt D, Thornton C, Tracy S, Homer C (2021) 'Modelling the cost of place of birth: a pathway analysis', *BMC Health Services Research*, 21, pp 1–11.

Scatliffe N, Casavant S, Vittner D, Cong X (2019) 'Oxytocin and early parent-infant interactions: a systematic review', *Int J Nurs Sci*, Sep 12 6(4):445-453. doi: 10.1016/j.ijnss.2019.09.009. PMID: 31728399; PMCID: PMC6838998.

Schmied V, Beake S, Sheehan A, McCourt C, Dykes F (2011) 'Women's perceptions and experiences of breastfeeding support: a metasynthesis', *Birth*, Mar 38(1):49-60. doi: 10.1111/j.1523-536X.2010.00446.x. Epub 2010 Dec 23. PMID: 21332775.

Scurry SI (2021) *The Breastfeeding Experience of Mothers in Postnatal Hospital Environments: An Ethnographic Study*, Doctoral dissertation, University of Technology, Sydney.

Shelton DC (2012) 'Man-midwifery history: 1730–1930', *Journal of Obstetrics and Gynaecology*, 32(8), 718–723. https://doi.org/10.3109/01443615.2012.721031. Accessed 6 June 2024.

Shimomura M, Morita Y, Hirai, Y (2017) 'Comparative research of childcare systems between Finnish Neuvola Service Design with Japanese services', Proceedings of the IASDR, pp 1883–1894.

Silva LAT, de Oliveira MIC, da Costa ACC, Morais Dos Santos SF, da Gama SGN, Fonseca VM (2022) 'Factors associated with infant formula supplementation in Brazilian hospitals: a cross-sectional study', *J Pediatr* (Rio J), Sep-Oct 98(5):463-470. doi: 10.1016/j.jped.2021.12.009. Epub 2022 Feb 25. PMID: 35227658; PMCID: PMC9510795.

Silva OLO, Rea MF, Sarti FM, Buccini G (2021) 'Cost-effectiveness analysis of Baby-Friendly Hospital Initiative in promotion of breast-feeding and reduction of late neonatal infant mortality in Brazil', *Public Health Nutr.* Jun 24(8):2365-2375. doi: 10.1017/S1368980020001871. Epub 2020 Jul 20. PMID: 32686631; PMCID: PMC10195532.

Smith J (2017) 'Markets in mothers' milk: Virtue or vice, promise or problem', *Making Milk: The Past, Present, and Future of Our Primary Food*, pp 117–138.

Smith, PM (1978) 'Mothers, babies, and the mothers and babies movement: Australia through depression and war', *Journal of Social History*, 12(2), pp 261–2.n.

Smith PM (1993) 'Mothers, babies, and the mothers and babies movement: Australia through depression and war', *Social History of Medicine*, 6(1), pp 51–83.

Smith J, Cattaneo A, Iellamo A, Javanparast S, Atchan M, Gribble K, Hartmann B, Salmon L, Tawia S, Hull N, Linkson M, Blake M, Elliott-Rudder M (2018) *Review of effective strategies to promote breastfeeding: an evidence check rapid review brokered by the Sax Institute for the Department of Health*, Sax Institute, Ultimo NSW, https://www.saxinstitute.org.au/publications/review-effective-strategies-promote-breastfeeding/. Accessed 10 June 2024.

'So, will you do it for your country?', *The Age*, 15 May 2004, https://www.theage.com.au/national/so-will-you-do-it-for-your-country-20040515-gdxur4.html. Accessed 29 April 2024.

Strathearn L, Mamun AA, Najman JM, O'Callaghan MJ (2009) 'Does breastfeeding protect against substantiated child abuse and neglect? A 15-year cohort study', *Pediatrics*, Feb 123(2):483-93. doi: 10.1542/peds.2007-3546. PMID: 19171613; PMCID: PMC2650825.

Summers A (1975) *Damned Whores and God's Police: the Colonization of Women in Australia*, Penguin, Australia.

Terashita S, Yoshida T, Matsumura K, Hatakeyama T, Inadera H; Japan Environment, Children's Study (JECS) Group (2023) 'Caesarean section and childhood obesity at age 3 years derived from the Japan Environment and Children's Study', *Sci Rep*.

Apr 21 13(1):6535. doi: 10.1038/s41598-023-33653-7. PMID: 37085536; PMCID: PMC10121560.

Tessier R, Cristo M, Velez S, Girón M, de Calume SZF, Ruiz-Paláez JG, Charpak Y, Charpak N (1998) 'Kangaroo mother care and the bonding hypothesis', *Pediatrics*, 102(2), pp e17–e17.

Tomori C (2023) 'Global lessons for strengthening breastfeeding as a key pillar of food security', *Frontiers in Public Health*, 11, 1256390.

Tomori C, Palmquist AE, Quinn EA eds (2017) *Breastfeeding: New Anthropological Approaches*, Routledge.

UNICEF (1989) 'The Convention on the Rights of the Child', https://www. unicef.org/child-rights-convention. Accessed 24 April 2024.

United Nations General Assembly (1948) 'Universal Declaration of Human Rights', 217 A (III), 10 December 1948, https://www.refworld.org/legal/resolution/unga/1948/en/11563. Accessed 3 April 2024.

United Nations General Assembly (1979) 'Convention on the Elimination of All Forms of Discrimination Against Women', 18 December 1979, United Nations, Treaty Series, vol. 1249, p. 13, http://www.un.org/womenwatch/daw/cedaw/cedaw.htm. Accessed 3 April 2024.

United Nations General Assembly (1989) 'Convention on the Rights of the Child', United Nations Treaty Series, vol. 1577, p. 3, 20 November 1989, https://www.refworld.org/legal/agreements/unga/1989/en/18815. Accessed 3 April 2024.

van Sadelhoff JHJ, van de Heijning BJM, Stahl B, Amodio S, Rings EHHM, Mearin ML, Garssen J, Hartog A (2018) 'Longitudinal variation of amino acid levels in human milk and their associations with infant gender', *Nutrients*, Sep 5 10(9):1233. doi: 10.3390/nu10091233. PMID: 30189593; PMCID: PMC6163519.

Vetcho S, Cooke M, Petsky H, Saito A, Ullman AJ (2022) 'Family-centred care change during COVID-19', *Nurs Crit Care*, May;27(3):460-468. doi: 10.1111/nicc.12766. Epub 2022 Mar 2. PMID: 35234320; PMCID: PMC9115396.

Victora CG, Bahl R, Barros AJ, França GV, Horton S, Krasevec J, Murch S, Sankar MJ, Walker N, Rollins NC; Lancet Breastfeeding Series Group (2016) 'Breastfeeding in the 21st century: epidemiology, mechanisms, and lifelong effect', *Lancet*, Jan 30 387(10017):475-90. doi: 10.1016/S0140-6736(15)01024-7. PMID: 26869575.

Vieira ACG, Bueno M, Harrison D (2020) 'Be sweet to babies: Use of Facebook as a method of knowledge dissemination and data collection in the reduction of neonatal pain', *Paediatric and Neonatal Pain*, 2(3), pp .93–100.

Woodward SC (2019) 'Fetal, neonatal, and early infant experiences of maternal singing', *The Oxford Handbook of Singing*, Oxford Handbooks Online, https://www.scribd.com/document/552627298/Sheila-C-Woodward-Fetal-Neonatal-and-Early-Infant-Experiences-of-Maternal-Singing. Accessed 6 June 2024.

World Health Organization (2014) Global nutrition targets 2025, Policy brief series, https://www.who.int/publications/i/item/WHO-NMH-NHD-14.2. Accessed 26 June 2024.

World Health Organization (2018) Nutrition and Food Safety, Ten steps to successful breastfeeding, https://www.who.int/teams/nutrition-and-food-safety/food-and-nutrition-actions-in-health-systems/ten-steps-to-successful-breastfeeding. Accessed 26 June 2024.

World Health Organization (2021) A 'First Embrace' after caesarian section is saving newborn lives in Viet Nam, https://www.who.int/westernpacific/news-room/feature-stories/item/a-first-embrace-after-caesarian-section-is-saving-newborn-lives-in-viet-nam#. Accessed 2 July 2024.

World Health Organization (2022) 'Marketing of breast-milk substitutes: national implementation of the international code', *Status Report 2022*, World Health Organization, Geneva. Accessed 4 July 2024.

World Health Organization (2023) *Monitoring health for the SDGs, Sustainable Development Goals 2023*, Global Report, https://www.who.int/publications/i/item/9789240074323. Accessed 6 June 2024.

World Health Organization (2023) 'World health statistics 2023: monitoring health for the SDGs', *Sustainable Development Goals*, https://cdn.who.int/media/docs/default-source/gho-documents/world-health-statistic-reports/2023/world-health-statistics-2023_20230519_.pdf. Accessed 6 June 2024.

World Health Organization (2024a) Maternal health, https://www.who.int/health-topics/maternal-health#tab=tab_1. Accessed 6 June 2024.

World Health Organization (2024b) Maternal mortality, https://www.who.int/news-room/fact-sheets/detail/maternal-mortality. Accessed 6 June 2024.

World Health Organization/Unicef (1990) 'Innocenti Declaration on the Protection, Promotion and Support of Breastfeeding', WHO/Unicef policymakers' meeting on 'Breastfeeding in the 1990s: A Global Initiative', SpedaledegliInnocenti, Florence, Italy, 30 July–1 August, 1990.

Ye J, Zhang J, Mikolajczyk R, Torloni MR, Gülmezoglu AM, Betrán AP (2016) 'Association between rates of caesarean section and maternal and neonatal mortality in the 21st century: a worldwide population-based ecological study with longitudinal data', *BJOG*, Apr 123(5):745-53. doi: 10.1111/1471-0528.13592. Epub 2015 Aug 24. PMID: 26331389; PMCID: PMC5014131.

Ylppo A (1954) 'Premature children; should they fast or be fed in the first days of life?' in *Annales Paediatriae Fenniae* vol. 1, no. 1, pp 99–104.

Zadoroznyj M, Brodribb WE, Young K, Kruske S, Miller YD (2015) 'I really needed help: what mothers say about their post-birth care in Queensland, Australia', *Women Birth*, Sep 28(3):246-51. doi: 10.1016/j.wombi.2015.03.004. Epub 2015 Apr 8. PMID: 25864129.

Acknowledgements

I would like to thank:

The women and babies who generously provided information and stories of their birthing and breastfeeding journeys, which inspired and encouraged me through to completion.
My colleagues for their support and faith,
My editor Brigid James who provided clarity when needed,
Jum, my life partner, for his generosity, patience and encouragement when sharing our story,
And my children and grandchildren, all a source of inspiration for a better future.